A Primer of Haematology

By the same Author

Clinical Investigation . . . By Means of Haematology
A Primer of Immunology
A Primer of Pathology

A Primer of Haematology

F. A. Ward, L.R.C.P.I., M.R.C.Path.

Senior Pathologist, Medical School, University of Natal; Consultant, Natal Institute for Immunology; formerly Deputy Medical Director, Natal Blood Transfusion Service; Pathologist, South African Institute for Medical Research

London : Butterworths

ENGLAND: BUTTERWORTH & CO. (PUBLISHERS) LTD.
LONDON: 88 Kingsway, WC2B 6AB

AUSTRALIA: BUTTERWORTH & CO. (AUSTRALIA) LTD.
SYDNEY: 20 Loftus Street
MELBOURNE: 343 Little Collins Street
BRISBANE: 240 Queen Street

CANADA: BUTTERWORTH & CO. (CANADA) LTD.
TORONTO: 14 Curity Avenue, 374

NEW ZEALAND: BUTTERWORTH & CO. (NEW ZEALAND) LTD.
WELLINGTON: 49/51 Ballance Street
AUCKLAND: 35 High Street

SOUTH AFRICA: BUTTERWORTH & CO. (SOUTH AFRICA) (PTY.) LTD.
DURBAN: 33/35 Beach Grove

Suggested U.D.C. Number: 616·15

ISBN 0 407 62506 2

2868
5.15

Printed in Great Britain by
Western Printing Services Ltd., Bristol

Contents

Preface

The success of *A Primer of Pathology* and *A Primer of Immunology* has induced Butterworths to request *A Primer of Haematology* which I herewith supply. As in the companion books, my object has been to tell the essentials of the story in as little space as possible. To give too much detail not only obscures the subject, it bores the reader which is worse.

To achieve brevity, I have omitted much physiology that is usually included in books on haematology and in my descriptions of disease processes, I have stressed only those points which are of importance in diagnosis. Throughout the book, I have, with few exceptions, avoided mentioning the more complicated tests and procedures and as far as possible I have been modest in regard to all laboratory tests. This was done, not only for the sake of brevity, but also because the vast majority of doctors, for one reason or another, cannot make use of these complicated and expensive tests.

To illustrate many points, I have made use of Clinical protocols most of which have been taken, with kind permission of the publishers, from *Clinical Investigation by Means of Haematology* (London: Butterworths). The cases presented in these protocols are, as far as medical cases can be, typical. I hope, therefore, that they will prove interesting and educational to the beginner.

Because of the ease with which a biopsy of the blood can be taken and because of the ease with which a blood count can be done, there seems to me no reason why a general practitioner should not be his own specialist as far as haematology is concerned. Yet many of them seem to fight shy of it. This is perhaps because haematology has developed a mystique which frightens the timid. I trust that this little book will help to dissolve any such mystique.

It is with pleasure that I acknowledge my indebtedness to my secretary, Vivien Morgan, who typed the manuscript, and I would like to thank the staff of Butterworths for their help in the production of this book.

F. A. WARD

1—Anaemia

DEFINITION

A patient is said to have anaemia when, while being in normal fluid balance, his haemoglobin concentration is below normal for that patient. There are two important points about this definition which are often not realized and which therefore require to be stressed.

(1) The importance of individual normality

The normal range of haemoglobin concentration for males at sea level is from 13·5 to 18·0 g per cent. An individual male, whose normal haemoglobin concentration is 18·0 g per cent may, as a result of a haemorrhage, present himself to the doctor with a haemoglobin concentration of 15·0 g per cent. Such a person is anaemic even though his haemoglobin level falls within the normal range. He deserves the same attention and treatment as a person whose haemoglobin level fell from 14·0 g per cent to 11·0 g per cent.

Furthermore, when we say that the normal haemoglobin concentration for males is from 13·5 g per cent to 18·0 g per cent, we are merely stating the near extremes of results found in a large number of normal males. In fact 95 per cent of normal males will be found to have haemoglobin values within these limits; there are, however, still 5 per cent of normal males who will have levels outside these limits. Thus a given male patient with a haemoglobin value of, say, 12·5 g per cent might be perfectly normal even though this value is below the lower limit of normal.

(2) The importance of normal fluid balance

A patient with a gastric ulcer may, as a result of chronic haemorrhage, have a haemoglobin concentration of, say, 12·0 g per cent. If now he has an attack of severe vomiting he will suffer dehydration and this will have the effect of raising his haemoglobin concentration

1

to perhaps 14·0 g per cent which is within the normal range. This patient, none the less, has anaemia; that it is complicated and obscured by another condition does not alter the fact. Dehydration is thus a common cause of misleading laboratory results and it undoubtedly explains many apparently conflicting reports.

Hardly less important, and causing the opposite effect, is over-hydration. In such conditions as nephritis, chronic liver disease and heart failure, there is an increase in plasma volume. This has the effect of diluting the haemoglobin, the concentration of which is therefore lowered. But this is not anaemia although anaemia often occurs in these conditions as well.

The interpretation of a haemoglobin result

From what has been said, we see that a person may have a haemo-globin concentration which is within the normal limits and he may still be anaemic. Furthermore, he may have a haemoglobin concen-tration below the normal limit and yet not be anaemic. It is apparent, therefore, that the results of a haemoglobin estimation must be read in the light of the clinical features of the case. What has been said about haemoglobin results applies equally to the packed cell volume (PCV) and the red cell count.

The clinical recognition of anaemia

There is only one clinical sign of anaemia worth mentioning and that is pallor. Pallor may be immediately apparent in the skin but this is often misleading, especially in dark-skinned races. It should be sought particularly in the mucous membranes of the mouth and conjunctivae. With experience it is possible to become proficient in assessing the colour of these membranes, but even with the most experienced there will always be a great number of doubtful cases. If, of course, an obvious cause for anaemia is found, for example profuse haemorrhage, then anaemia may be diagnosed with complete confidence.

The laboratory recognition of anaemia

The laboratory recognition of anaemia depends on either a haemoglobin or a PCV estimation. There is little to choose between the accuracy of either of these tests. In practice both should be done so that the mean corpuscular haemoglobin concentration (MCHC), which gives important additional information, can be calculated. In the past, red cell counts were frequently done; these give the same kind of information as the haemoglobin and PCV estimations. They were, however, tedious, time consuming and inaccurate and for these reasons they fell largely into disuse. More recently, however, with the advent of electronic particle counters, it has become possible to do an accurate red cell count quickly and without tedium. With the red cell count and the PCV the mean corpuscular volume (MCV) can be calculated. This is a useful index in certain doubtful cases.

The laboratory investigation of anaemia (initial steps)

In this section the phrase 'full blood count' is used to mean a haemoglobin estimation, a PCV estimation (with MCHC) and a survey of a suitably stained blood film.

All patients suspected of having anaemia should have a full blood count. The haemoglobin estimation and PCV will confirm (or refute) the clinical impression, and the MCHC will, if below 30 per cent provide proof of hypochromic anaemia. From the MCHC and the appearance of the red cells on the film, the anaemia is assigned to one or other of the following categories. This is the morphological classification of anaemia.

(1) Macrocytic   (normochromic or hypochromic).
(2) Normocytic   (normochromic or hypochromic).
(3) Microcytic   (normochromic or hypochromic).

The assignment of a case of anaemia to its proper category in the morphological classification is the first step in reaching the ultimate diagnosis. Other useful information can sometimes be obtained from a survey of the smear. The main points are listed in Table 1.

TABLE 1

Finding	Significance
Increased diffuse polychromasia and and reticulocytosis	Regenerative anaemia e.g. haemolytic anaemia
Absence of polychromasia and reticulocytes	Aregenerative anaemia e.g. aplastic anaemia
Spherocytes and schistocytes	Haemolytic anaemia
Burr cells, helmet cells and triangular cells	Micro-angiopathic haemolytic anaemia
Target cells	Haemoglobinopathy e.g. Mediterranean anaemia
Sickle cells	Sickle cell anaemia
Megaloblasts	Megaloblastic anaemia
Giant myeloid cells	Megaloblastic anaemia
Punctate basophilia	Lead poisoning and other conditions
Malarial parasites	Malaria
Leucocytosis	Infection, leukaemia, etc.

THE PATHOGENESIS OF ANAEMIA

There are scores of causes of anaemia, yet all these arise by one or more of the following easily remembered pathogenetic mechanisms: (1) haemorrhage; (2) excess haemolysis (haemolytic anaemia); (3) marrow failure.

The importance and frequency of these mechanisms

Haemorrhage

Apart from trauma, haemorrhage is a concomitant of a great number of diseases many of which are exceedingly common. Amongst these are peptic ulcer, gastro-intestinal cancer, haemorrhoids, hiatus hernia, menorrhagia, cirrhosis of the liver and the complications of pregnancy and childbirth.

Excess haemolysis

There is a tendency to consider this mechanism uncommon, yet, when one reflects on the widespread distribution of malaria, the haemoglobinopathies and haemolytic disease of the newborn, the importance of excess haemolysis as a cause of anaemia begins to be realized. Furthermore, excess haemolysis occurs in a number of more or less common diseases in which it is overshadowed by other features of the disease.

Marrow failure

First among the causes of marrow failure is malnutrition, and in this connection it is sufficient to say that three-quarters of the world's population are under-fed.

The multifactorial origin of anaemia

In practice it is found that anaemia often arises from more than one of the above pathogenetic mechanisms. Thus, anaemia in a given patient may be caused partly by marrow failure (due to malnutrition), partly by haemorrhage (due to hookworms) and partly by excess haemolysis (due to malaria). Even in such a distinct clinical entity as Addison's pernicious anaemia, the anaemia is caused partly by marrow failure and partly by excess haemolysis.

It is therefore wise always to look for more than one pathogenetic mechanism in a given patient. Nevertheless, in the majority of patients it will be found that one mechanism predominates and that this is often, but by no means always, apparent on clinical examination.

Erythropoiesis in anaemia

In any of the above-mentioned pathogenetic mechanisms of anaemia the erythropoiesis may be one or other of two well-defined types, normoblastic or megaloblastic. In normoblastic erythropoiesis there is an orderly development of the red cells, the nucleus and the cytoplasm developing *pari passu*. In megaloblastic erythropoiesis there is disorder in that while the cytoplasm develops reasonably normally, the nucleus is delayed in its maturation. It is this asynchronism, or lack of correspondence between cytoplasmic and nuclear development, which is the hall-mark of megaloblastic erythropoiesis. In addition the red cells are larger than normal, giant myeloid cells are formed and usually there is a deficiency in platelet production.

While normoblastic erythropoiesis occurs in the vast majority of patients with anaemia, there is an important group of anaemias characterized by megaloblastic erythropoiesis. Basically these arise as a result of vitamin B_{12} deficiency, folic acid deficiency or a combination of both. However, these deficiencies arise in a wide variety of conditions (*see* pages 36 and 40).

The recognition of megaloblastic erythropoiesis

When megaloblastic erythropoiesis is taking place in the bone marrow, suggestive, sometimes pathognomonic, changes occur in the peripheral blood. These changes include macrocytosis, many of the macrocytes being oval rather than round, and marked poikilocytosis, large pear-shaped poikilocytes being particularly suggestive. Often giant myeloid cells appear in the blood. The multilobed neutrophil, also known as the macropolycyte, is the most common and it, too, is highly suggestive. Usually there is a decrease in the number of platelets.

Sometimes megaloblasts are seen in the ordinary blood film but more often they are found in a film prepared from the buffy layer. When they are identified the presence of megaloblastic erythropoiesis in the bone marrow is certain. The film appearance, however, gives no indication of the *cause* of the megaloblastic erythropoiesis. If megaloblasts are not found in the peripheral blood it may be necessary to examine the bone marrow.

2—The Anaemia of Haemorrhage

Of the three pathogenetic mechanisms of anaemia, haemorrhage is the easiest to understand. It is obvious that if a person loses a considerable quantity of blood, he will become anaemic; but the functional activity of the bone marrow must not be forgotten. This organ is capable of tremendous hyperplasia with the result that anaemia following a mild haemorrhage is cured spontaneously. Haemorrhage is conveniently divided into two forms, acute and chronic. This is an imprecise division which has no scientific basis, yet it is useful because in typical cases the clinical and blood pictures of the two are quite different.

ACUTE HAEMORRHAGE

Acute haemorrhage means a sudden loss of a sizeable quantity of blood. Typical examples include the haemorrhage from wounds, the haemorrhage following the complications of pregnancy and child-birth, the haemorrhage from benign and more especially malignant ulcers and the voluntary periodic haemorrhage of blood donors. There are three points about acute haemorrhage which are commonly overlooked and therefore require to be stressed.

(1) In acute haemorrhage, it is not the anaemia but the shock which gives rise to anxiety. A normal person can lose a pint of blood in a matter of minutes and be almost unaware of any ill effect. Blood donors do this regularly. But the loss of two or more pints in the same period of time will lead to shock and it is this which constitutes the real danger. It is important to grasp this point because in the treatment of acute haemorrhage valuable time is often wasted while waiting for compatible blood for a blood transfusion. What is needed immediately is plasma to combat the shock; blood transfusion can follow later if required.

(2) Immediately after an acute haemorrhage the patient's haemoglobin concentration is substantially the same as it was before the haemorrhage occurred. It is not until the plasma volume is restored (by a draft from the interstitial tissue) that the haemoglobin level reaches its low point. This process may require 24 hours or more. What has been said about haemoglobin concentration applies equally to the PCV and the red cell count; hence any of these estimations is misleading immediately after an acute haemorrhage. The severity of the case must be decided on clinical grounds, especially on the blood pressure.

(3) The final point about acute haemorrhage which is often forgotten is the situation in regard to iron. A moderately severe haemorrhage, for example 2 pints of blood, means that the patient has lost about 500 mg of iron. In regenerating the blood lost, the patient will therefore draw about 500 mg of iron from his stores which, in a normal person, amounts to about 1,000 mg. The stores will thus suffer a measure of depletion. Consideration should therefore be given to replenishing the iron stores. In mild cases it is not necessary, in severe cases it is mandatory, in no case is it an urgency.

The blood picture following acute haemorrhage

The blood picture following acute haemorrhage will vary depending on the time that has elapsed since the haemorrhage has occurred. As already stated, the haemoglobin level may be normal or only slightly depressed immediately after the haemorrhage. The most prominent features in the blood count are a thrombocytosis and a leucocytosis. The leucocytosis takes the form of a neutrophilia, and with this, primitive myeloid cells may appear in the circulation. This is known as a shift to the left. The red cells show evidence of active marrow function, namely, increased diffuse polychromasia, reticulocytosis and possibly macrocytosis. After some weeks, if the iron stores have been depleted by the haemorrhage, the red cells will become microcytic and hypochromic (*see* Clinical protocol 1).

CHRONIC HAEMORRHAGE

Chronic haemorrhage means a gradual loss of blood over a period of weeks, months, or even years. Unlike the acute variety it is likely to be overlooked by both patient and doctor because of its insidious onset and course.

Chronic haemorrhage does not lead to shock but to profound anaemia. Typical examples of this kind of haemorrhage occur in lesions of the gastro-intestinal tract such as peptic ulcer, cancer of the stomach, hiatus hernia, cancer of the colon, cancer of the rectum and haemorrhoids. In women, menorrhagia is the most important form of chronic haemorrhage.

In the treatment of the anaemia due to chronic haemorrhage it is important to remember that the plasma volume of the patient is essentially normal; hence, if transfusion is considered it is better to transfuse packed cells rather than whole blood. This avoids over-burdening the heart which is possibly already weakened having laboured in a condition of partial anoxia for some time. Having treated the cause of the haemorrhage, or sometimes even before treating it, it is necessary to provide the patient with adequate iron. This is best given by mouth; seldom is it necessary to resort to parenteral administration. Iron treatment must be continued not only until the patient's haemoglobin level is satisfactory but for at least 2 months thereafter. This latter precaution is necessary in order to replenish the depleted iron stores.

The blood picture in chronic haemorrhage

The red cells are hypochromic and microcytic; they show aniso-cytosis, poikilocytosis and increased diffuse polychromasia. The white cells and platelets vary from case to case. The essential point to remember is that the anaemia is hypochromic, microcytic and regenerative in type.

This blood picture, if found in an adult male, is almost patho-gnomonic of chronic haemorrhage. In a woman of child-bearing age, in addition to chronic haemorrhage, it is often due to dietary iron deficiency aggravated by menstruation (sometimes menorrhagia) and pregnancy. In infants and children it is most often due to dietary deficiency of iron aggravated by the increased requirements of growth. A similar, but not necessarily identical, blood picture is found in Mediterranean anaemia; some cases of infection and the rare pyridoxine-responsive anaemia of which I have yet to see an example (*see* Clinical protocol 2).

The treatment of the anaemia of chronic haemorrhage

The haemorrhage should be stopped. This often requires a surgical operation and as such the problem is outside the scope of this book. But before an operation is performed, and in those cases where it is not indicated, it is usually necessary to proceed immediately to the treatment of the anaemia *per se*.

In severe cases a blood transfusion is required. The transfused blood provides not only fully haemoglobinized red cells but also iron and clotting factors. The red cells will be destroyed in a few weeks, but the iron will persist in the body and will be available for erythro-poiesis later. In this connection it is useful to remember that each half litre of blood contains about 250 mg of iron. The clotting factors in the transfused blood may be of great value should the patient be deficient in this regard.

In milder cases, the anaemia of chronic haemorrhage may be treated as iron deficiency anaemia, a topic which will be considered later.

Clinical protocol 1. The Anaemia of acute haemorrhage

A middle-aged woman was brought to hospital because of a compound fracture of the femur with severe haemorrhage.

Haemogram

Haemoglobin	9·6 g%	White cell count	17,000/mm³
		Neutrophils	70%
PCV	30%	Monocytes	3%
		Lymphocytes	27%
MCHC	32%	Eosinophils	0%
		Basophils	0%

The red cells are normochromic and normocytic; they show anisocytosis, occasional macrocytes and increased diffuse polychromasia. There is a neutrophilia with a shift to the left. The platelets are greatly increased in number.

Comment

This is a typical haemogram of acute haemorrhage. It is not possible to say precisely how severe the anaemia is because two pieces of information are not available, that is, it is not known what period of time elapsed between the injury and the collection of the blood specimen, and it is not known what the patient's normal haemoglobin level is. With regard to the first point, if the blood specimen was collected within a few hours of the injury, it may be expected that the haemoglobin level will fall further as fluid moves from the interstitial tissue into the circulation. With regard to the second point, if the patient's normal haemoglobin level is 11·5 g per cent, then at the present time she is only 1·9 g per cent below her normal value. If, how-ever, her normal value is 14·0 g per cent, then she already has a 4·4 g per cent, haemoglobin deficit; the patient's condition must therefore be assessed on clinical grounds.

The occasional macrocytes and the polychromasia reflect

9

increased activity of the erythroid series in the bone marrow which is a compensatory phenomenon. There is no satisfactory explanation for the behaviour of the white cells and the platelets, it seems that acute haemorrhage is a general marrow stimulus.

Clinical protocol 2.   Chronic haemorrhage

A woman aged 57 years was admitted to hospital because of weakness, pallor and abdominal pain.

Haemogram

Haemoglobin	6·8 g%	White cell count	11,000/mm³
		Neutrophils	48%
PCV	24%	Monocytes	5%
		Lymphocytes	45%
MCHC	28%	Eosinophils	2%
		Basophils	0%

The red cells are hypochromic and microcytic; they show anisocytosis, poikilocytosis and increased diffuse polychromasia. There is a slight lymphocytosis. The platelets are normal in number and appearance.

Comment

This is a typical haemogram of chronic haemorrhage. It could also be due to nutritional iron deficiency, but the complaint of abdominal pain suggested an abnormality of some sort in the abdomen.

As there was no history of haemorrhage, the stool was tested for occult blood. It yielded a negative result. The gastro-intestinal tract was then examined radiologically but again no abnormality was detected.

Undeterred by these negative results, the surgeon in charge of the patient performed a laparotomy and discovered an advanced carcinoma of the caecum. It was therefore concluded that the anaemia was due to chronic haemorrhage from this carcinoma of the caecum.

Apart from illustrating chronic haemorrhage, this case shows how laboratory tests and radiographs can, on occasions, mislead. Even the haemogram, which told so much truth, had a misleading element in the lymphocytosis for which no cause could be found.

The anaemia in this case was treated by blood transfusion before, during and after the operation.

3—The Anaemia of Excess Haemolysis

THE SYNDROME OF HAEMOLYTIC ANAEMIA

The essence of haemolytic anaemia is a destruction of red cells which is in excess of the capacity of the bone marrow to produce red cells. Normally the life span of the red cells is about 120 days but in cases of haemolytic anaemia it is reduced to 20 days or less. Various causes of this shortened life span will be considered later; here we are concerned with the effects of this excessive destruction in the body. First we shall deal with the physiopathological changes which occur, then we shall discuss the clinical features.

Haemolytic jaundice

Excessive destruction of red cells implies excessive catabolism of haemoglobin and this in turn implies excessive formation of un-conjugated bilirubin. There is therefore a tendency for the serum unconjugated bilirubin to rise and thus cause jaundice; this is known as haemolytic or prehepatic jaundice. The liver, however, increases its activity in regard to bilirubin excretion, hence the rise in the serum bilirubin is usually moderate or slight and often insufficient to cause clinical jaundice. But in newborn infants, because of the immaturity, jaundice is prominent.

Unconjugated bilirubin is insoluble, hence it does not give the direct reaction with diazo reagent. The characteristic reaction in the haemolytic syndrome is a negative direct, but a positive indirect, reaction in the van den Bergh test. Being insoluble, unconjugated bilirubin is bound to albumen for the purpose of transportation in the blood. This explains why it is not excreted by the kidneys and thus why haemolytic jaundice is described as acholuric.

Although not soluble in water, unconjugated bilirubin is soluble in lipid. It is therefore liable to enter the brain and, should its con-centration exceed the power of albumen to bind with it, it may do so

11

thus causing irreversible brain damage; this is known as kernicterus. It never occurs in obstructive jaundice and hardly ever in haemolytic jaundice in adults, but in newborn babies it is the dreaded complication of haemolytic disease.

Because of the increased concentration of bilirubin in the bile, pigment gallstones may form and these may lead to attacks of biliary colic. Such stones are not visible by plain radiography of the abdomen, indeed they may be difficult to demonstrate even with the use of contrast media. Increased bilirubin in the intestine results in increased formation of urobilinogen. Some of this urobilinogen is excreted in the stool, where it is often called stercobilinogen, and some of it is reabsorbed to be excreted in the urine. Increased faecal and urinary urobilinogen are therefore features of the haemolytic syndrome.

Haemoglobinaemia, Haemoglobinuria, Haemosiderinuria

If the destruction of the red cells occurs intravascularly, haemoglobin is liberated in the plasma; this is called haemoglobinaemia. Such free haemoglobin seems to be dealt with by three distinct mechanisms. Firstly it is taken up by the haptoglobins; when these are saturated it is taken up by the serum albumen and at this stage the Schuum's test becomes positive. Finally, when this mechanism is exhausted, the haemoglobin is excreted in the urine thus causing haemoglobinuria.

Some of the haemoglobin which is excreted into the glomerular filtrate is reabsorbed by the renal tubular cells where it is converted into haemosiderin. This has been demonstrated convincingly in postmortem sections of the kidney which have been specifically stained. Subsequently this haemosiderin is excreted in the urine where again it can be detected by the prussian blue reaction.

Compensatory phenomena

With the excessive destruction of red cells, there is a compensatory hyperplasia of the bone marrow. This change can be directly observed by an examination of the marrow and it is reflected in the peripheral blood by the appearance of increased numbers of reticulocytes and polychromatic cells. These, and other newly formed cells, are generally larger than normal cells; hence there is a tendency towards macrocytosis, and sometimes the blood film shows frank macrocytosis. In many cases this shift to the left of the red cells is accompanied by a leucocytosis, with a shift to the left of the neutrophils. The leucocytosis is often due to an intercurrent infection but sometimes it seems to be due to haemolysis *per se*.

The aplastic crisis

Occasionally, far from being hyperplastic, the bone marrow becomes aplastic; this is known as the aplastic crisis. It may interrupt the usual course of the disease at any time and lasts about 2 weeks. It is recognized by an increase in the degree of anaemia together with a decrease in the degree of jaundice. The aplastic marrow is reflected in the peripheral blood by an absence of reticulocytes and polychromatic cells and a reduction in the number of white cells and platelets The cause of such a crisis is unknown; it is believed that in some instances it is brought about by infection.

Sites of the excessive red cell destruction

Reference has already been made to intravascular haemolysis but, malaria excluded, in most cases the excess haemolysis occurs extravascularly. It is then of more than academic interest to know where precisely it is taking place.

With the introduction of the radioactive chromium (^{51}Cr) method for labelling red cells, it has become possible to determine the site of excess haemolysis *in vivo* with considerable accuracy. Sometimes it is found that the excess haemolysis is occurring in both the liver and the spleen, but in other cases it is occurring in the spleen only. It is these cases that often benefit greatly from removal of the spleen.

Relative deficiencies of folic acid and vitamin B_{12}

The excessive bone marrow activity, which may be five or six times greater than normal, will obviously involve a greater utilization of iron, folic acid and vitamin B_{12}. Because the iron resulting from the destruction of red cells is re-usable, there is usually no shortage of this commodity; hence haemolytic anaemias are seldom hypochromic in type. If, however, there is prolonged haemoglobinuria or haemosiderinuria, or if there is a deficiency of iron for some other reason, then the anaemia will be hypochromic in type.

This favourable situation with regard to iron does not obtain to either folic acid or vitamin B_{12}; hence in patients who are poorly stocked with these essential factors, a relative deficiency may occur in which event the anaemia will be megaloblastic in type. In poorly or undernourished patients, therefore, it is wise to make sure that there is no nutritional deficiency which would complicate what is already probably a complicated condition.

The clinical features of the haemolytic syndrome

The clinical features of the haemolytic syndrome vary from mild to severe. Sometimes the process is so rapid that it may suggest an acute internal haemorrhage, but more often it is an unobtrusive or a totally silent process. In many cases the features of the haemolytic syndrome are completely overshadowed by the features of the condition which caused the haemolytic process.

They consist essentially of pallor, rigors, jaundice, enlargement of the spleen and pain. The pain may be in the abdomen, back or limbs; sometimes the chief complaint is of a severe headache. With the exception of the jaundice, which is often absent, and the enlargement of the spleen, which is often not palpable, there is little among these clinical features to suggest a diagnosis of haemolytic anaemia. This explains why it is so seldom recognized at the bedside.

There are, however, two ways in which the syndrome may be brought to light. Firstly, it may be noticed that a patient treated by blood transfusion for anaemia of unknown origin fails to maintain a satisfactory haemoglobin level. This feature, in the absence of haemorrhage, is very strong evidence of the haemolytic syndrome. Secondly, and more usually, it is brought to light by a routine blood count.

The blood picture in haemolytic anaemia

The anaemia may be mild or severe; the red cells are nearly always normochromic and normocytic. Sometimes, if the process is severe of if there is a relative deficiency of folic acid, the cells will be macrocytic. Rarely, if there is a concomitant iron deficiency for any reason, the cells will be hypochromic and microcytic. Anisocytosis of some degree is always present but it is of little help in diagnosis. Poikilocytosis is much more helpful. Small darkly staining cells suggest spherocytes which not only mark the case as a haemolytic anaemia but place it in the category of spherocytic haemolytic anaemia. Not infrequently the irregularities in the shape of the cells immediately suggest micro-angiopathic haemolytic anaemia. Curved elongated banana-shaped cells suggest sickle cell anaemia while an abundance of target cells will suggest Mediterranean anaemia. Except during the aplastic phases of a haemolytic process, the red cells show evidence of regeneration, that is, reticulocytosis and increased diffuse polychromasia.

The white cells may be normal, but often there is a neutrophilia with a shift to the left. This may be due to an intercurrent infection which often occurs, or to the haemolysis *per se*. The presence of giant myeloid cells will suggest a relative folic acid deficiency.

The platelets vary; in the micro-angiopathic group of haemolytic anaemias they are typically reduced in number.

The investigation of the haemolytic syndrome

Once the syndrome of haemolytic anaemia has been recognized, the problem of its cause must be solved. Various schemes have been proposed for this purpose but no one scheme is applicable in all cases. As so often happens in clinical medicine, each patient must be investigated as a separate problem. In malaria for example, which is probably the commonest cause of the haemolytic syndrome in the world as a whole, the malaria itself may be recognized before the haemolytic syndrome. As this is an ultimate diagnosis the question of investigating the haemolytic syndrome is irrelevant. The same applies to cases of leukaemia which are complicated by the haemolytic syndrome.

In obscure cases, apart from the blood count, the direct Coombs test is probably the best preliminary step. This test will divide all haemolytic anaemias into Coombs negative and Coombs positive types. The former is represented mainly by the hereditary haemolytic anaemias, the latter by the auto-allergic haemolytic anaemias. Further investigation will depend on the circumstances that obtain in the particular patient under consideration.

Family history in haemolytic anaemia

As many cases of haemolytic anaemia are inherited, it is important to enquire into the family history whenever this condition is suspected in a patient. It is important, not only for the purpose of establishing the diagnosis more firmly in the patient under consideration, but also because it may bring to light other cases. Should such cases be discovered, it seems only right and fair that the significance of their defect should be explained to them in easily understood language. I have found, even among illiterate people, that they readily understand these things and are highly appreciative of the advice given.

Hereditary spherocytosis is the best example of a haemolytic anaemia determined by a simple dominant gene. This mode of inheritance implies that one or other parent must also possess the gene, and, because it is dominant, must manifest the condition to a greater or lesser extent. It is important to remember that it may be manifested to a lesser extent; for example, parents of a patient may insist that they enjoy good health but examination of the blood film will reveal that one or other has spherocytosis. Such subclinical cases are not uncommon. The mode of inheritance also implies that, on average, half the patient's siblings and half the patient's children will also have the condition in a clinical or subclinical form.

The inheritance of sickle cell anaemia presents a little difficulty.

15

For practical purposes it may be regarded as a disease due to a recessive gene. It is true that the gene expresses itself in the heterozygote and is thus entitled to be called dominant or co-dominant, but the expression in the heterozygote is not sickle cell anaemia but sickle cell trait, a condition which gives rise to symptoms only in abnormal conditions of low oxygen tension such as high flying in a non-pressurized aircraft. It is only in the homozygous state, that is, when the gene is inherited from *both* parents, that sickle cell anaemia occurs in ordinary conditions of living.

Viewed as a recessive gene, it is all the more sinister as the trait cannot be recognized by potential husbands and wives. Thus the gene is propagated and if two such genes occur together in the same person, sickle cell anaemia is the result. Therefore, as with all diseases determined by recessive genes, sickle cell anaemia occurs more commonly, but not exclusively, in association with consanguinity.

THE CAUSES OF HAEMOLYTIC ANAEMIA

Malaria

Malaria is probably the commonest cause of haemolytic anaemia. Not very long ago it was estimated that malaria caused 1 death every 10 seconds, but things have no doubt improved since then. It is usually associated with tropical and subtropical regions but with increasing population movements this localization is no longer valid. The disease, however, can flourish only where the anopheline mosquito flourishes, though occasional examples of transmission by blood transfusion occur.

It is suspected from its clinical features, notably fever, rigors, generalized body pains, headache and enlargement of the spleen; the suspicion is confirmed by microscopic examination of the blood film. When the blood specimen is sent to the laboratory it is important to mention the suspicion of malaria, otherwise the parasites are easily overlooked.

The disease is treated with quinine, chloroquine, atebrine or paludrine, any of which, if given in adequate amounts, will bring about marked relief in 24–48 hours. In cases of doubt, treatment should be started without waiting for the laboratory report (*see* Clinical protocol 3).

Haemoglobinopathy

Haemoglobinopathy, with which is included Mediterranean anaemia, is probably the second most common cause of haemolytic anaemia. The various haemoglobinopathies, like malaria, have a regional distribution but, for the reason given for malaria, this distribution is not to be regarded as absolute. Haemoglobinopathy may be suspected from the clinical history or from a routine blood count, it is confirmed by haemoglobin electrophoresis (*see* Clinical protocols 4 and 5 and *Figure* 1).

Drugs and other chemicals

The number of drugs and other chemicals which are known to cause haemolytic anaemia (and other haematological disorders) is enormous. This being so, no examination of a patient is complete until the question of drug-taking and exposure to noxious chemicals has been explored.

In some instances the haemolytic anaemia is caused by the direct toxic action of the drug on the red cells (for example phenylhydrazine), in others the toxic effect of the drug is enhanced by a deficiency of the enzyme glucose-6-phosphate dehydrogenase in the red cells (for example primaquine) and in still others the drug acts through an auto-allergic mechanism (this will be mentioned under auto-antibodies).

Sometimes the diagnosis of members of this group of haemolytic anaemias is easy as, for example, when a severe haemolytic syndrome, complete with haemoglobinuria, follows the ingestion of broad beans.* But more often it is impossible, on clinical grounds, to do more than suspect the condition. A blood count will probably reveal the features of haemolytic anaemia, and Heinz bodies, if sought and found, will provide strong confirmatory evidence.

Iso-antibodies

Iso-antibodies constitute a major cause of haemolytic anaemia. The most important of the iso-antibodies are anti-C (of the ABO system) and anti-Rh_0 (of the rhesus system). Other iso-antibodies are occasionally responsible for the disease. Although haemolytic disease of the newborn due to anti-C is possibly more common than that due to anti-Rh_0, the latter is by far the more serious.

The disease is suspected when jaundice occurs in the first 24 hours of life; it is confirmed in the laboratory by observing a materno-foetal blood group incompatibility and by a positive direct Coombs test on the baby's red cells. It is treated by simple transfusion or, in more severe cases, by exchange transfusion. Kernicterus, due to excess unconjugated bilirubin in the blood, is the main complication.

* Broad beans are not usually looked upon as poisonous, but for many people in this world there is no other name for them.

Auto-antibodies

Auto-antibodies must be distinguished from iso-antibodies. Auto-antibodies are antibodies which a person develops and which are reactive against his own tissues, in this context against his own red cells. These antibodies often arise in association with some other morbid condition, notably malignant lymphoma, lupus erythematosus and drug poisoning, but in some 50 per cent of cases there is no such association.

Auto-allergic haemolytic anaemia, as the disease is now called, may be suspected on clinical grounds. That it is a haemolytic anaemia is shown by the blood count, but to establish that it is auto-allergic in origin requires serological tests, especially the direct Coombs test. The treatment consists in treating the associated condition which, when present, often dominates the clinical picture. The others, called idiopathic, often respond well to steroid therapy.

Micro-angiopathy

A number of diseases in which lesions of small blood vessels occur are often associated with a peculiar form of haemolytic anaemia which is distinguished by the adjective micro-angiopathic. The blood picture in these cases is quite characteristic. Apart from the almost constant features of haemolytic anaemia, the red cells show a remarkable degree of poikilocytosis in which burr cells, helmet cells, triangular cells and spherocytes are prominent. There is strong evidence to show that the lesions in the blood vessels physically injure the red cells resulting in their distortion and subsequent premature destruction. Among the many diseases which are known to give rise to this train of events the most important are malignant hypertension, thrombotic thrombocytopenic purpura, renal cortical necrosis and acute nephritis. Micro-angiopathic haemolytic anaemia is diagnosed by recognizing the characteristic appearance of the blood film (*see* Clinical protocol 6).

Myelophthisis

Myelophthisic anaemia, as its name suggests, is due to a lesion in the bone marrow. This lesion is most commonly a secondary carcinoma but it may be a reticulum cell sarcoma, myeloma, myelofibrosis, Hodgkin's disease or primary xanthomatosis; in one of my cases it was a retinoblastoma. The pathogenesis of the anaemia was originally thought to be due to replacement of the normal bone marrow by one or other of these space-occupying lesions. This theory is no longer tenable; it never really was. More recently it has been shown that in many cases the pathogenesis of the anaemia is excess haemolysis, hence the inclusion of myelophthisic anaemia here; the blood picture further justifies this inclusion. It is often described as leuco-erythroblastic anaemia, a description which would fit most cases of haemolytic anaemia. The outstanding feature of the blood film is the presence of an unexpectedly large number of normoblasts in the face of a slight to moderate degree of anaemia. Sometimes fairly characteristic tear-drop shaped poikilocytes may be seen.

This form of anaemia is seldom, if ever, diagnosed by purely clinical means. It is usually brought to light by a routine blood count. Like megaloblastic anaemia, myelophthisic anaemia is not an ultimate diagnosis. Once its presence has been established, the question of its cause must be pursued (*see* Clinical protocol 7).

Hereditary spherocytosis

Hereditary spherocytosis is due to a genetically determined defect of the red cells. These cells assume a spherical shape and are thus readily trapped and destroyed by the spleen. That is the immediate cause of the anaemia. Removal of the spleen cures the disease but does not alter the defect in the red cells. The disease is suspected on clinical examination by noting paroxysmal jaundice, splenic enlargement and possibly ulceration of the legs. It is confirmed by a blood count on the patient, which will establish the presence of spherocytic anaemia, and blood counts on the patient's near relatives, which will establish its hereditary character. Spherocytes have an increased osmotic fragility, a characteristic which can be demonstrated by the test of that name (*see* Clinical protocol 8).

Infections

A great number of infections, both bacterial and viral, may cause haemolytic anaemia. In these cases, however, it is usually the infection which dominates the clinical picture, the haemolytic anaemia being an incidental finding. Among the bacteria which may cause haemolytic anaemia, *Clostridium welchii* deserves special mention. Infection with this organism may follow abortion.

Miscellaneous

Haemolytic anaemia occurs irregularly in a great variety of other conditions including chronic renal disease, chronic liver disease, ovarian tumours, incompatible blood transfusion, intravenous infusion of water. It also occurs in vitamin B_{12}, folic acid and iron deficiency, but in these cases it is seldom prominent.

19

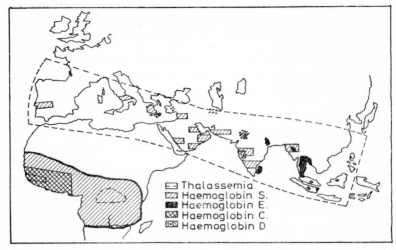

Figure 1. The geographical distribution of the most common haemoglobin variants

Clinical protocol 3. Malaria

A man aged 45 years had been complaining of headache, backache and pains in the limbs for about a week. The only note-worthy findings on physical examination were a slight pyrexia and an enlargement of the spleen.

Haemogram

Haemoglobin	11·8 g%	White cell count	15,000/mm³
		Neutrophils	60%
PCV	36%	Monocytes	17%
		Lymphocytes	20%
MCHC	33%	Eosinophils	2%
		Basophils	1%

The red cells are normochromic and normocytic; they show anisocytosis, slight poikilocytosis and increased diffuse polychromasia. There is a monocytosis. Platelets are normal in number and appearance.

Comment

An acute infection of one sort or another is suggested by the clinical history of the case. This, together with the enlargement of the spleen, would naturally indicate the need for a blood count.

The haemogram shows a mild normochromic normocytic regenerative anaemia. This immediately suggests a haemolytic process. The only other clue in the haemogram is the monocytosis.

Monocytosis is not a common finding in practice. It occurs irregularly in a number of conditions including enteric fever, brucellosis, subacute bacterial endocarditis, tuberculosis, glandular fever, Hodgkin's disease, monocytic leukaemia and such tropical diseases as malaria, kala-azar and trypanosomiasis. It is therefore a signal to the haematologist to search for malarial parasites. When this was done, they were indeed found.

When malaria is suspected, a blood film should be made and specific treatment started at once without waiting for the result from the laboratory. This precaution will save perhaps many hours' delay during which the fate of the patient may be decided. There is no doubt that, as with diphtheria, the sooner treatment is started, the better is the prognosis.

Clinical protocol 4.   Mediterranean anaemia

A baby aged 3 months was taken to hospital because of extreme pallor. Prior to this, the patient had been treated for iron deficiency, but there had been no improvement. On examination, in addition to the pallor, a moderate enlargement of the spleen was detected. The baby, though a caucasoid, had a suggestively mongoloid appearance. The mother could not see this, but she admitted that many of her neighbours had commented on it.

Haemogram

Haemoglobin	2·6 g%	White cell count	86,000/mm³
		Neutrophils	39%
PCV	13%	Monocytes	0%
		Lymphocytes	52%
MCHC	22%	Eosinophils	4%
		Basophils	0%
		Myelocytes	4%
		Blast cells	1%

The red cells appear normocytic and markedly hypochromic; they show anisocytosis, poikilocytosis, increased diffuse polychromasia and occasional macrocytes. Target cells were seen also. More than 300 normoblasts were seen in the course of the differential count. The white cells show a shift to the left. The platelets appear slightly reduced in number.

Comment

The clinical data, were it not for the failure of iron treatment, would suggest iron deficiency anaemia. This failure to respond to iron is important, as it brings to light many cases of Mediterranean anaemia. Mediterranean anaemia is one of the few diseases which may be recognized at a glance, because sometimes the patient presents a typical mongoloid appearance. In this case, however, it was not pronounced. The haemogram, together with electrophoresis of the parents haemoglobin, confirmed the diagnosis. Another approach to the diagnosis is to estimate the serum iron and total iron binding capacity (TIBC). In this condition the serum iron is raised and the TIBC is saturated.

Blood transfusion is the mainstay of treatment. If there is evidence of hypersplenism, as there sometimes is, splenectomy may be considered.

Clinical protocol 5.   Sickle cell anaemia

Three days before admission to hospital, an Indian man 20 years of age was awakened one night by severe pain in the lower limbs. Apart from headache, there was no other symptom. On arrival at hospital nothing abnormal could be found in the limbs but an enlargement of the spleen was discovered in the course of the physical examination.

Haemogram

Haemoglobin	11·8 g%	White cell count	16,000/mm³
		Neutrophils	80%
PCV	36%	Monocytes	3%
		Lymphocytes	17%
MCHC	33%	Eosinophils	0%
		Basophils	0%

The red cells are normochromic and normocytic; they show anisocytosis, poikilocytosis and increased diffuse polychromasia. Target cells are also present. There is a neutrophilia; Platelets are normal in number and appearance.

Comment

The discovery of an enlarged spleen demands a blood count as a preliminary step towards the solution of the problem. The blood count, showing as it does a normochromic normocytic regenerative anaemia, immediately suggests excess haemolysis

22

as the pathogenetic mechanism. The neutropenia may be due to the haemolysis *per se*, or it may be due to an undetected infection. There is nothing in the haemogram to suggest the cause of the haemolysis except the target cells. These cells are found in Mediterranean anaemia and a number of haemoglobinopathies. Further investigations indicated in this case are therefore a test for sickling and haemoglobin electrophoresis.

The test for sickling was positive; this indicated either sickle cell anaemia or sickle cell trait. Haemoglobin electrophoresis confirmed the presence of sickle cell anaemia.

Enlargement of the spleen is not to be regarded as typical of sickle cell anaemia; indeed far from being enlarged, the spleen may be atrophic. A bizarre clinical picture in itself demands a blood count.

Clinical protocol 6.   Micro-angiopathic haemolytic anaemia

A man aged 50 years, who was known to have had high blood pressure for a number of years, was admitted to hospital because of heart failure. Examination of his optic discs showed the presence of papilloedema.

Haemogram

Haemoglobin	10·1 g%	White cell count	12,000/mm^3
		Neutrophils	68%
PCV	30%	Monocytes	5%
		Lymphocytes	25%
MCHC	34%	Eosinophils	2%
		Basophils	0%

The red cells are normochromic and normocytic; they show anisocytosis, poikilocytosis and increased diffuse polychromasia. Helmet cells, burr cells, spherocytes and triangular forms were observed among the red cells. The white cells are normal in appearance. The platelets are reduced in number.

Comment

The clinical data place the diagnosis as malignant hypertension. The haemogram is typical of micro-angiopathic haemolytic anaemia. It is generally believed that the root cause of the anaemia is the physical injury to the red cells by abnormal blood vessels. This injury results in their grotesque distortion and subsequent destruction.

The syndrome of micro-angiopathic haemolytic anaemia was

made prominent by M. C. Brain, J. V. Dacie and D. O'B. Hourihane in the *British Journal of Haematology* (1962, **8,** 358). The following list, taken from their article, shows the variety of conditions in which they found this blood picture.

Thrombotic thrombocytopenic
  purpura
Malignant hypertension
Renal cortical necrosis
Microscopic polyarteritis nodosa
Acute glomerulonephritis

Systemic lupus
  erythematosus
Cancer of the stomach
Cancer of the lung
Cancer of the prostate

Clinical protocol 7.   Myelophthisic anaemia

A male aged 74 years was admitted to hospital because of difficulty in passing urine. This had been present for at least 12 months. There was no other significant feature in the patient's history.

Haemogram

Haemoglobin	9·5 g%	White cell count	11,000/mm^3
		Neutrophils	71%
PCV	29%	Monocytes	8%
		Lymphocytes	21%
MCHC	33%	Esinophils	0%
		Basophils	0%

The red cells are normochromic and normocytic. They show anisocytosis, slight poikilocytosis and increased diffuse polychromasia. In the course of the differential count 8 normoblasts were seen. There is a slight neutrophilia with a shift to the left. The platelets are normal in number and appearance.

Comment

Difficulty in passing urine in a patient of this age is nearly always due to enlargement of the prostate gland, and this enlargement is most often due either to benign adenomatous hyperplasia or adenocarcinoma.

The haemogram shows a moderate normochromic normcytic regenerative anaemia, and this immediately suggests excess haemolysis as the pathogenetic mechanism. The presence of the normoblasts in such a moderate anaemia is highly suggestive of a space-occupying lesion in the bone marrow, and, in view of the history, this lesion is most likely to be a secondary carcinoma from a primary growth in the prostate gland.

Such a diagnosis would be confirmed by an estimation of the serum acid phosphatase, a radiological examination of the skeleton and, most importantly, by a histological examination of the prostate.

There is no adequate explanation to account for the appearance of normoblasts in these cases. They do not invariably appear, but when they do they constitute a clue which should never be disregarded.

Clinical protocol 8. Hereditary spherocytosis

A boy aged 17 years, who complained of malaise following what was said to be influenza, was admitted to hospital for investigation. He was found to have pallor, a slightly yellow tinge in his sclera and a moderately enlarged spleen.

Haemogram

Haemoglobin	9·5 g%	White cell count	12,000/mm^3
		Neutrophils	68%
PCV	27%	Monocytes	4%
		Lymphocytes	28%
MCHC	35%	Eosinophils	0%
		Basophils	0%

The red cells are normochromic and normocytic; they show anisocytosis, spherocytosis and increased diffuse polychromasia. There is a slight neutrophilia. Platelets are normal in number and appearance.

Comment

It is not uncommon for patients with hereditary spherocytosis to present themselves in this rather misleading way. Furthermore, although it is a hereditary disease, it often remains latent until adulthood. The pallor, the jaundice and the enlarged spleen together indicate haemolytic anaemia; the haemogram confirms this and shows it to be spherocytic haemolytic anaemia. The hereditary nature of the condition is ascertained by family studies. In this case, the father of the patient was found to have spherocytes in his blood although he had no complaints.

The pathogenesis of the disease is reasonably well understood. As a result of a genetically determined metabolic defect of the red cells, spherocytes instead of biconcave cells appear in the blood. These are quickly trapped and destroyed in the spleen. When the process of destruction is in excess of that which can be compensated for by the bone marrow, haemolytic anaemia is inevitable.

Removal of the spleen will cure the disease but it requires fine clinical judgement to know when to advise it. In general, it may be said that if the disease is interfering materially with normal life, splenectomy is indicated. The operation, of course, does not cure the defect in the red cells.

4—The Anaemia of Marrow Failure

Marrow failure is the third pathogenetic mechanism of anaemia. It is also the most complicated. Many of the anaemias considered under this heading here are classified as deficiency or nutritional anaemias in other works. This difference should not lead to confusion.

Marrow failure is defined here as a condition where, in the absence of excess haemolysis and haemorrhage, the marrow fails to perform its function of supplying red cells in adequate quantity and quality.

THE CAUSES OF MARROW FAILURE

The following are the three main causes of marrow failure.
(1) Malnutrition.
    (a) General malnutrition
    (b) Iron deficiency
    (c) Folic acid deficiency
    (d) Vitamin B_{12} deficiency
(2) Inhibition of the marrow.
    (a) Infection
    (b) Renal failure
    (c) Drug and chemical poisoning
    (d) Idiopathic (aplastic anaemia)
(3) Endocrine deficiency.
    (a) Hypothyroidism
    (b) Addison's disease

The diagnosis of marrow failure

If, in a case of anaemia, excess haemolysis and haemorrhage can be excluded, then the patient must have marrow failure. Marrow failure, however, is not an adequate diagnosis, but as a provisional diagnosis it is a useful step in the further clinical and laboratory investigation of the patient.

Because of the heterogeneous collection of conditions included under this heading, it is not possible to say more about the diagnosis of the group as a whole. This much, however, may be said: in haemorrhage and haemolytic anaemia, evidence of red cell regeneration (increased polychromasia and increased reticulocytes) is expected and is usually prominent. In the above conditions it is often, but not always, absent.

Erythropoiesis in marrow failure

Erythropoiesis in marrow failure may be normoblastic or megaloblastic. Rarely, as in cases of aplastic anaemia, there may be no evidence of erythropoiesis at all. In all but two of the above-mentioned causes of marrow failure, the erythropoiesis is usually normoblastic in type. The two exceptions are folic acid deficiency and vitamin B_{12} deficiency, in which the erythropoiesis is megaloblastic.

Megaloblastic anaemia

Megaloblastic anaemia results from megaloblastic erythropoiesis which, it may be said for practical purposes, is due to folic acid deficiency, vitamin B_{12} deficiency, or a combination of both. The circumstances in which the deficiencies occur will be considered later.

Megaloblastic erythropoiesis gives rise to the formation of macrocytes. These are large, often oval, red cells which have a shortened life span. There is therefore a haemolytic element in megaloblastic anaemias. As well as macrocytes, large pear-shaped poikilocytes are often present and are of diagnostic significance. Megaloblasts are sometimes found in the ordinary blood film, but there is a much greater chance of finding them in a film made from the buffy layer. This is a very useful and rather neglected procedure in the diagnosis of megaloblastic anaemia. Often, however, it is necessary to examine the bone marrow to establish the presence of megaloblastic erythropoiesis beyond doubt.

The white cells also are affected in megaloblastic anaemia. The characteristic findings are a leucopenia, which is essentially a neutropenia, a shift to the left of the neutrophils, and the presence of giant myeloid cells. These cells, often in the form of multilobed neutrophils and called macropolycytes, are highly suggestive but not quite pathognomonic of megaloblastic anaemia. The platelets are often reduced in number.

Megaloblastic erythropoiesis is inefficient; many red cells are destroyed before they are fully formed. Such ineffective erythropoiesis is the major cause of the anaemia in these cases.

In temperate climates megaloblastic anaemia is due to vitamin

28

B_{12} deficiency (pernicious anaemia) in some 90 per cent of cases. In tropical climates it is due to folic acid deficiency (malnutrition) in about 90 per cent of cases.

THE ANAEMIA OF GENERAL MALNUTRITION

General malnutrition, in the sense in which it is used here, refers to cases such as those seen in the German concentration camps, in the Warsaw Ghetto and those which are still seen in vast areas of the tropics. It is essentially protein malnutrition, and since the days of Whipple it has been known that protein deficiency is a cause of anaemia. It is idle, at this stage, to bother about which of the amino acids are needed for blood formation; a person with general malnutrition requires first class protein, that is meats, fish, poultry, eggs and milk. When we say that three-quarters of the world's population are undernourished, we must keep in mind that protein malnutrition is the heart of the problem. But malnutrition is seldom specific. A person who is deficient in one element of the diet is likely to be deficient in others. This will become apparent when we consider the aetiology of the condition.

Malnutrition and infection

Although examples of 'pure' malnutrition occur, the condition is nearly always complicated by infection. Indeed, malnutrition leads to infection and infection leads to malnutrition; both lead to anaemia. This important concept is shown diagrammatically as follows:

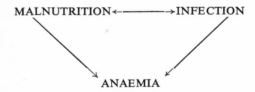

Because of this association between malnutrition and infection, the use of antibiotics, and possibly a surgical operation (the drainage of an abscess), may be essential in the treatment of the anaemia of malnutrition.

The aetiology of general malnutrition

The aetiology of general malnutrition is largely a social problem; nevertheless, because of its importance to the doctor, it will be outlined here. Poverty is the most obvious and most frequent cause of malnutrition. It is not, however, distinct from apathy and ignorance; indeed, the three often go together.

Even among the most impoverished communities, there is usually sufficient means to obtain the necessary carbohydrate in the form of rice, maize, cassava, potatoes and others; but these, while they satisfy hunger and supply energy, do not provide a basis for blood manufacture. What is needed are meats, fish, poultry, eggs and milk, all of which are expensive articles of the diet. This explains why a person suffering from gross malnutrition may still deny that he is the slightest way hungry.

Poverty, as a cause of malnutrition, is usually complicated by ignorance, thus it is quite common to find that what little money is available is misused. Carbonated drinks, for example, are often bought instead of milk and what protein food is available is often taken by the adults who need it less than the children.

Not infrequently, the practitioner comes across malnutrition in reasonably well to do persons. Old widows and widowers living alone are often too apathetic to bother about preparing proper meals for themselves. They live mainly on bread and tea, and this eventually leads to malnutrition and anaemia. Fortunately, there are various proprietary food concentrates available which will at least ease, if not completely solve, their problem.

Alcoholism is another, often overlooked, cause of malnutrition. In a word, the alcoholic prefers his alcohol to his food and often this preference is so pronounced that malnutrition results.

Finally, there are those who, for religious, traditional or other reasons, deprive themselves of food. Some African people, for example, will not allow their young daughters to eat eggs. In this way, the girls are deprived of a rich source of both protein and iron.

The morphological types of anaemia

The anaemia of general malnutrition is usually normochromic and normocytic in type. The red cells may become thinner and their diameters may increase and for these reasons they may appear on the stained film as hypochromic macrocytes. But in the vast majority of cases they have a normal MCV and a normal MCHC. Sometimes the anaemia may be truly macrocytic, the macrocytes arising from macronormoblastic or, more uncommonly, megaloblastic erythropoiesis. Sometimes the anaemia is hypochromic and microcytic and sometimes it appears to be a mixture of the two when it is referred to as dimorphic anaemia.

There is often a neutrophilia due to an intercurrent infection.

Diagnosis

The diagnosis of the anaemia of general malnutrition should present little difficulty in the vast majority of cases. The general appearance of the patient is usually suggestive, and a simple enquiry into the dietary habits and the amount of money which is spent on food is often revealing.

Treatment

From what has been said already, the treatment of this form of anaemia should be apparent. It is usual to advise patients to take a balanced diet. This advice is excellent when it can be understood and when it can be followed, but here is where the economic factors must not be forgotten. Nothing is more frustrating than trying to cure anaemia among the poor. Protein and iron are generally found in the more expensive foods, but liver and kidney are notable exceptions which are often overlooked. Unfortunately, they are not always acceptable. Lettuce is probably the best source of folic acid but even lettuce is sometimes expensive. It is probably true to say that iron, folic acid and vitamin B_{12} can be obtained more cheaply from the chemist than from the butcher or greengrocer. Iron tablets or tonics should not be given unless specifically indicated as it tends to depress the appetite and thus make matters worse.

A factor, sometimes neglected, is the infection which is so often present. Any such infection should be adequately treated because until such time as it is cured, the other measures will not have the desired effect (*see* Clinical protocol 9).

Clinical protocol 9. General malnutrition

A male aged 48 years was admitted to hospital because of ascites and oedema of the feet. He gave a history of flatulent dyspepsia which extended over a period of 7 to 8 years. More recently, he complained of muscular weakness and great loss of energy. The patient was pale, emaciated and had a slight enlargement of the spleen.

Haemogram

Haemoglobin	9·5 g%	White cell count	5,000/mm³
		Neutrophils	48%
PCV	30%	Monocytes	7%
		Lymphocytes	45%
MCHC	32%	Eosinophils	0%
		Basophils	0%

The red cells are normochromic and normocytic; they show slight anisocytosis and slight poikilocytosis. There is a mild neutropenia. The platelets are normal in number and appearance.

Comment

In looking through my records for a case to illustrate general malnutrition, I find I have plenty to choose from. Kwashiorkor would perhaps have provided the most telling example, yet I finally decided on this, a case of portal cirrhosis, not only because it presents certain instructive clinical features, but also because it serves to illustrate malnutrition in the more ordinary circumstances of western European life.

The anaemia of liver cirrhosis may arise from all three of the basic pathogenetic mechanisms. Haemorrhage may result from oesophageal varices; excess haemolysis, though seldom prominent, is coming to be recognized as a common feature in liver disease. Marrow failure, resulting from malnutrition, probably occurs in all cases sooner or later.

The malnutrition in these cases may be due to dietary deficiency coupled with malabsorption and it may be in regard to protein, folic acid or vitamin B_{12}. In the present case, the present case, the evidence is in favour of marrow failure due to protein malnutrition.

THE ANAEMIA OF IRON DEFICIENCY

The term 'iron deficiency anaemia' is ambiguous. It could be used, and indeed it has been used, to mean any of the following.

(1) Anaemia due to deficient iron in the diet.
(2) Anaemia due to deficient iron absorption.
(3) Anaemia due to deficient iron utilization.
(4) Anaemia due to haemorrhage.

When using the term, it is important to remember its various connotations and the liability of the listener or the reader to getting the wrong one. It is preferable therefore to use one or other, whichever is applicable, of the above phrases whenever possible.

Sometimes 'iron deficiency anaemia' is used synonymously with 'hypochromic anaemia'. This is incorrect; to do so is to confuse the aetiology with the microscopic appearance of the red cells.

Anaemia due to deficient iron in the diet

A full diet contains about 15–20 mg of iron per day. Allowing for the fact that only about 10 per cent of this is absorbed, we see that such a diet provides only 1·5 – 2 mg of iron per day. This amount is just about the same as the normal daily loss of iron. For men this is adequate, but for women who have to meet the demands of menstruation and pregnancy, the situation is critical. Iron deficiency anaemia, due to lack of iron in the diet, must therefore be suspected in all anaemic women especially those who have had several pregnancies.

When is this most likely to occur?

Anaemia due to deficient iron in the diet is most likely to occur in any of the following conditions.
(1) During pregnancy (especially in multipara, in the lower classes, in multiple pregnancies).
(2) During infancy (especially if premature, if twins, if mother was iron deficient).
(3) During periods of rapid growth (especially in the lower classes).

What foods contain iron?

Pre-eminent among the foods which contain iron is one which is often neglected, namely liver. Other important sources are kidney, meats and eggs; green vegetables are largely over-rated in this regard. Less obvious sources of iron are water (from deep wells but only in certain areas) and the iron from utensils used in cooking. With the increasing use of glass and aluminium cooking utensils, this latter source is waning. There is no iron in beer (it gives beer a bad taste) and insignificant amounts in wine.

Anaemia due to deficient iron absorption

Many factors influence the absorption of iron including HCl and vitamin C which enhance it, and phytic acid and phosphates which depress it. Nevertheless, anaemia due to deficient absorption of iron is uncommon and for practical purposes may be said to occur only in association with steatorrhoea.

Anaemia due to deficient iron utilization

Deficiency of iron utilization is found typically in Mediterranean anaemia but it also occurs in some cases of infection, renal failure and other conditions. As the defect in these cases is in the utilization of iron, the administration of iron does not help matters. For research purposes, these cases are investigated by the radio-iron utilization test.

Anaemia due to haemorrhage

Anaemia due to haemorrhage is discussed on page 6.

The diagnosis of dietary iron deficiency anaemia

The early clinical manifestations of iron deficiency are vague and unimpressive. They consist of tiredness, dry brittle hair and brittle finger nails. The patient often does not mention these to the doctor unless specifically questioned. Strangely enough, she often mentions them to the chemist or hairdresser. Angular stomatitis, atrophic glossitis and koilonychia occur much later, if indeed they occur at all. A peculiar form of dysphagia, part of the Plummer–Vinson syndrome is rare; I have never seen it.

Contrary to what might be expected, there seems to be no direct relation between the severity of the symptoms and the haemoglobin level. Thus many of my patients complain of extreme tiredness with a haemoglobin level of 10 g per cent, yet one of my patients had no symptoms whatsoever with a haemoglobin level of 7 g per cent and he was a long-distance runner.

The disease is most common in women and this is doubtlessly because the physiological functions of a woman (pregnancy and menstruation) make a demand for iron which the diet often fails to satisfy. That explains why a wife may have iron deficiency anaemia while her husband, living on the same diet, is a full-blooded man. In many cases, however, the diet is obviously deficient in iron and a few simple enquiries will often reveal this.

The ultimate diagnosis of iron deficiency anaemia depends on laboratory investigations. A hypochromic microcytic type of anaemia is sufficient evidence for most doctors to start treatment, but it is not the final proof. Serum iron and TIBC estimations may be required to distinguish the hypochromic anaemia of iron deficiency from the hypochromic anaemia of infection (*see* page 44), and the best, but most uncomfortable, test of all is an examination of the bone marrow for haemosiderin.

The treatment of anaemia due to deficiency of dietary iron

Common sense would suggest that the diet should be corrected in regard to its deficiency; this undoubtedly ought to be done. But by itself it is hardly adequate. Tablets containing ferrous sulphate are the commonly recommended method. The treatment should be continued for at least 2 months after the patient's haemoglobin has reached a satisfactory level, this is to ensure that the iron stores will be replenished.

This regimen sounds simple enough, but often problems arise. The crux of the matter is that the therapeutic dose of iron is toxic for many patients. They suffer, to a greater or lesser extent, from gastro-intestinal disorders such as anorexia, nausea, vomiting and constipation. One of my patients had an attack of vomiting after a single tablet, which continued intermittently for 6 or 7 hours, by which time he was vomiting bile. Needless to say, he is no longer a patient of mine. After I tried some iron tablets myself I began to see why some patients prefer their anaemia to its treatment.

The basic problem is that, as only a small fraction of any iron compound is absorbed, large toxic doses have to be given. If the percentage of iron absorbed could be increased, then the total dose could be reduced accordingly. This seems to have been achieved in the product Ferromyn-S (ferrous succinate and succinic acid) in which, because of greater absorption, a very small dose of elemental iron (37 mg per tablet) is incorporated.

Another way around the difficulty is to use parenteral iron. This method has many advocates, but it suffers from the obvious disadvantage that it requires a visit to or from the doctor. In addition, it is not without danger. I have used it with comparatively few patients, but because of one or two serious side reactions, I avoid it if it is at all possible (*see* Clinical protocol 10).

Clinical protocol 10. Nutritional iron deficiency anaemia

A girl aged 17 years was admitted to hospital because of swollen legs. The swelling had been present for about 1 week. No other symptoms were offered, but on direct questioning the patient admitted to having experienced weakness, tiredness, brittle finger nails and brittle falling hair. Examination revealed a poorly nourished girl with oedema of the sacrum and lower limbs. The jugular veins were distended, the heart was enlarged and there was a double mitral murmur. The clinical diagnosis was heart failure.

Haemogram

Haemoglobin	8·9 g%	White cell count	10,000/mm³
		Neutrophils	75%
PCV	31%	Monocytes	2%
		Lymphocytes	19%
MCHC	29%	Eosinophils	4%
		Basophils	0%

The red cells are hypochromic and microcytic; they show

anisocytosis, poikilocytosis and increased diffuse polychromasia. The white cells are normal. The platelets are normal in number and appearance.

Comment

The clinical diagnosis of heart failure was undoubtedly correct, and the laboratory diagnosis of microcytic hypochromic anaemia provided at least a contributory cause of the heart failure. The problem thus resolved itself into finding the cause of the anaemia.

In the vast majority of cases hypochromic microcytic anaemia is due to iron deficiency caused either by chronic haemorrhage or by a deficiency of iron in the diet. Appropriate enquiries should therefore be made to find out which of these two was concerned in this case.

On further questioning of the patient, nothing emerged which would suggest chronic haemorrhage. Even her menstrual periods were scanty. Questions concerning her diet, however, brought forth the most interesting information. The patient subsisted mainly on rice, bread and tea. It was therefore reasonable to conclude that this was a case of nutritional iron deficiency anaemia.

THE ANAEMIA OF FOLIC ACID DEFICIENCY

Folic acid

Folic acid is found in a variety of foodstuffs especially in green leafy vegetables; hence its name. Lettuce, cabbage and spinach are particularly valuable sources. It is heat-labile, therefore a large proportion of the folic acid in food is destroyed during cooking. Lettuce, which is eaten raw, is thus more valuable than cabbage, which is always cooked. As a haemopoietic agent, folic acid is probably inactive until it is converted into folinic acid and for this conversion vitamin B_{12} appears to be important. It is possible that vitamin C also plays a part in the conversion.

The anaemia

Folic acid is necessary for normal red cell development (normoblastic erythropoiesis), and in its absence, the bone marrow reverts to a more primitive and less efficient form of red cell development known as megaloblastic erythropoiesis. The anaemia of folic acid deficiency is therefore macrocytic normochromic in type. An associated iron deficiency will of course render it hypochromic. Folic acid deficiency manifests itself also in the myeloid cells which are often bigger than normal. Representatives of these so-called giant myeloid cells are often found in the peripheral blood; the large multinucleated neutrophil being the most typical example. Platelets are usually reduced in number, but this feature is not prominent in the majority of cases.

When is folic acid deficiency most likely to occur?

Folic acid deficiency is most likely to occur in the following circumstances.

(1) *Malnutrition.* Malnutrition is by far the most common cause of folic acid deficiency. It is particularly likely to occur during pregnancy and infancy among the poorer classes. But even among the well to do, folic acid deficiency during pregnancy is occasionally encountered.

(2) *Malabsorption.* Malabsorption of folic acid occurs in some patients with coeliac disease and adult sprue.

(3) *Cirrhosis of the liver.* Folic acid deficiency is sometimes associated with cirrhosis of the liver. The precise nature of the association is not clear; in many patients it may be a nutritional defect.

(4) *Defective utilization of folic acid.* This occurs as a result of administering folic acid antigonists. These include a number of drugs which are used in the treatment of epilepsy. If folic acid is given to such patients, the anticonvulsant drug need not be withdrawn. Infection also interferes with the action of folic acid and this is the most common cause for failure of a folic acid deficient patient to respond to treatment.

(5) *Haemorrhage and excess haemolysis.* These, by causing an increase in erythropoiesis in the bone marrow, may precipitate a mild folic acid deficiency. The erythropoiesis, therefore, instead of being normoblastic in type, would become megaloblastic. These examples show clearly the importance of considering the patient as a whole and thus avoiding the blindness which results from adherence to water-tight classifications.

The diagnosis of folic acid deficiency

Folic acid deficiency is seldom, if ever, diagnosed on purely clinical grounds, though it may be suspected when severe anaemia occurs in pregnancy. In the vast majority of cases, the diagnosis is first seriously suggested by a routine blood count when the typical, but not pathognomonic, blood picture is seen. If megaloblasts are not found in the ordinary blood film, they may be detected in a buffy layer prepared from the peripheral blood. If they are still not detected, it may be necessary to examine the bone marrow. Thus it will be established that the anaemia is megaloblastic in type. Such information, in the presence of a compatible clinical picture, is all that is necessary in most cases. Sometimes, however, further more elaborate investigations are required.

The histamine loading or FIGlu excretion test

In the normal course of metabolism, histamine is converted into urocanic acid, formamine-glutamic acid (usually called FIGlu), and finally glutamic acid which is excreted in the urine. In the absence of folic acid, the final conversion of FIGlu cannot occur; hence this product accumulates and is excreted in the urine where it can be detected by spectrophotometric or electrophoretic methods.

In the FIGlu excretion test, this metabolic pathway is stressed by giving the patient a large dose, usually 15 g of histamine. The patient then empties his bladder and the urine excreted in the following 8 hours is collected in a jar containing a few crystals of thymol and 5 ml of N HCl. The urine is then examined for FIGlu, which is greatly increased in patients with megaloblastic anaemia due to folic acid deficiency.

Some claim that the test is very valuable but false results have been reported in a variety of conditions, particularly pernicious anaemia, liver disease and pregnancy. Much experience is therefore required if the results are to be interpreted correctly.

Serum folic acid assay

In some circumstances a serum folic acid assay is advisable. This is the most sensitive indication of folic acid deficiency but is time consuming and tedious. For these reasons it is not generally available at the present time, but there are great hopes that it soon will be. The normal range for serum folate is from 6–21 ng/ml.

Tests for folic acid absorption

The serum folic acid level is measured before and again after the administration of a large dose of folic acid by mouth. Alternatively, the absorption of folic acid may be investigated by a test similar to the Schilling test but using radioactive folic acid instead of radioactive vitamin B_{12}. Neither of these methods is generally available. Fortunately, they are seldom required (*see* Clinical protocol 11).

Latent folic acid deficiency

Before leaving the problem of folic acid deficiency, it is necessary to point out that minor degrees of this deficiency which do not cause megaloblastic anaemia are very common in general hospital patients and probably also in the general public. Thus, while megaloblastic anaemia occurs in about 1 per cent of pregnant women, a minor degree of folic acid deficiency (as shown by a low serum folic acid level) occurs in up to 60 per cent. The precise significance of these subclinical cases is not yet known, but when they occur in association with diseases of unknown or doubtful aetiology, they are tantalizing and they certainly suggest that folic acid may take its place with protein and iron among the great deficiencies of the world. It may, of course, turn out that measurements of serum folic acid, as a criterion of folic acid deficiency, are too sensitive for practical purposes and that more reliance should be placed on red cell folate levels.

Clinical protocol 11. Folic acid deficiency

A woman aged 30 years, who was in poor financial circumstances and in the late months of her pregnancy, was admitted to hospital because of weakness and tiredness. On examination, marked pallor of her mucous membranes was noted.

Haemogram

Haemoglobin	3·0 g%	White cell count	5,000/mm³
		Neutrophils	60%
PCV	9%	Monocytes	7%
		Lymphocytes	28%
MCHC	33%	Eosinophils	5%
		Basophils	0%

The red cells are normochromic and macrocytic; they show marked anisocytosis, marked poikilocytosis, schistocytosis and increased diffuse polychromasia. Howell–Jolly bodies were seen also. The total and differential white cell counts are normal. The platelets appear to be reduced in number. Megaloblasts were detected in the buffy layer.

Comment

Megaloblastic anaemia of pregnancy is probably the commonest way in which folic acid deficiency manifests itself. It may present in various and often misleading ways, such as heart failure, accidental haemorrhage or pyrexia of unknown origin. There is thus no such thing as a 'typical' clinical presentation. Once the anaemia has been recognized, however, the subsequent blood count will suggest, if not expose, the megaloblastic nature of the condition. Often an examination of the buffy layer is required; seldom an examination of the bone marrow. Not infrequently, the blood picture is obscured by a concomitant iron deficiency.

Treatment consists of folic acid and attention to any infection which might be present. Because of the very low haemoglobin concentration, blood transfusion using packed cells is indicated, but, if labour is likely to begin within a day or two, then exchange transfusion offers the only hope of raising the haemoglobin concentration to a reasonable level in the time available.

THE ANAEMIA OF VITAMIN B_{12} DEFICIENCY

Vitamin B_{12}

Vitamin B_{12} is synthetized by various micro-organisms, notably *Streptomyces aurofaciens* and *S. griseus*; indeed, these organisms are used for the commercial production of the vitamin. Other organisms, notably *lactis* and *Lactobacillus leishmanii*, while requiring the vitamin for growth, are unable to synthetize it. These therefore are useful for assaying the vitamin. Vitamin B_{12} is found in liver, meat, eggs and to a lesser extent in milk and cheese. It is not found in vegetable foods.

Like folic acid, vitamin B_{12} is required for normoblastic erythro-poiesis and without it megaloblastic erythropoiesis occurs. It is probable that its essential action in this connection is to convert folic into folinic acid. The vitamin is also important in preserving the integrity of the central nervous system.

The absorption of Vitamin B_{12}

The absorption of vitamin B_{12} is dependent on the presence of an intrinsic factor in the gastric juice. Intrinsic factor is believed to be a mucoprotein; it is normally secreted by the gastric mucosa. Failure to secrete this factor results in Addison's pernicious anaemia. Vitamin B_{12} is absorbed in the lower part of the small intestine; hence disease in this area may also interfere with absorption.

When is the deficiency likely to occur?

(1) *Following atrophy of the gastric mucosa.* Due to atrophy of the gastric mucosa there is an absence of intrinsic factor which results in a deficiency of vitamin B_{12}. The precise cause of the gastric atrophy is not clear, but there is evidence that it is auto-allergic in origin and that this auto-allergy is genetically influenced. This is the essential pathogenesis of Addison's anaemia which is the commonest form of vitamin B_{12} deficiency.

(2) *Following surgical removal of the stomach.* As a result of a complete gastrectomy, there will be no intrinsic factor and hence no absorption of vitamin B_{12}. In practice, it is found that anaemia due to this mechanism takes years to develop; indeed the patient often dies before the anaemia has time to develop. This is because of the large stores of vitamin B_{12} in the liver.

(3) *Following intestinal abnormalities.* A variety of abnormalities of the intestinal tract have been known to lead to megaloblastic anaemia, some cases of which required vitamin B_{12} to cure; others required folic acid. These abnormalities include regional ileitis, intestinal stricture, intestinal resection, ileocolic fistula and blind loops. The mechanism by which these conditions produce megaloblastic anaemia varies. In some of them (blind loops) it is because of a change in the intestinal flora, the new bacteria competing with the host for vitamin B_{12}. Steatorrhoea in childhood and adults is also sometimes associated with megaloblastic anaemia, but it seems that folic acid deficiency is the main factor in these cases.

(4) *Following infestation with Diphyllobothrium latum.* This infestation has been given more attention than it deserves. It is fairly common in certain parts of Iceland and Finland, but only about 1 per cent of those infested develop megaloblastic anaemia. It appears that the worm simply competes with the host for the available vitamin B_{12}; it is thus said to be the purest form of vitamin B_{12} deficiency.

(5) *Following dietary deficiency.* It has already been said that vitamin B_{12} does not occur in vegetable foods. Then what about vegetarians? The Vegans are a tribe of strict vegetarians and they do not seem to suffer much from their dietary deficiency. I nearly always have one or two Vegans in my class and I cannot impress them with the importance of dietary vitamin B_{12}. Bernard Shaw, perhaps the most famous of all vegetarians, died at 94 years of age, and then because of a broken leg. I wish someone would explain all this to me; it's not only a puzzlement, it's an embarrassment.

Maybe this is the explanation. At the best of times only an exceedingly small amount of vitamin B_{12} is required and perhaps in the presence of abundant folic acid, even lesser amounts are needed. This might also explain, in part at least, why so few people with *Diphyllobothrium latum* infestation develop megaloblastic anaemia.

The clinical effects of vitamin B_{12} deficiency

The effects of vitamin B_{12} deficiency are manifested mainly in the blood, the alimentary tract, the peripheral nervous system, the spinal cord and the brain.

THE ANAEMIA OF MARROW FAILURE

(1) *The blood.* Pallor, weakness, fatigue, dyspnoea on exertion, perhaps a faint jaundice.
(2) *The alimentary tract.* Sore tongue (atrophic glossitis), loss of appetite, nausea, vomiting, diarrhoea.
(3) *Peripheral nerves.* Paraesthesia of hands and feet, unsteady gait, impaired superficial sensation.
(4) *Spinal cord.* Loss of vibration sense, Romberg's sign, ataxia, muscular spasticity, extensor plantar responses.
(5) *The brain.* Loss of memory, mental depression, irritability, sexual impotency, mania (*see* Clinical protocol 12).

Clinical protocol 12.   Pernicious anaemia

A man aged 60 years was admitted to hospital because of weakness, tiredness and breathlessness. It was not possible to ascertain the duration of these symptoms; they were certainly present for many months. On direct questioning, the patient admitted to numbness and tingling of his hands and feet and also of a slight soreness of the tongue. On examination, his conjunctivae were pale but there was no suggestion of jaundice.

Haemogram

Haemoglobin	5·0 g%	White cell count	4,000/mm³
		Neutrophils	35%
PCV	15%	Monocytes	7%
		Lymphocytes	54%
MCHC	33%	Eosinophils	4%
		Basophils	0%

The red cells are normochromic and macrocytic; they show anisocytosis, poikilocytosis, increased diffuse polychromasia and punctate basophilia. Occasional cells showing Howell–Jolly bodies were seen also. There is a neutropenia. Some macropolycytes were seen. The platelets appear to be reduced in number.

Comment

Many authorities say that the diagnosis of pernicious anaemia is a fairly easy task; I have never been able to verify this. The insidious nature of the disease, the fact that it occurs in older persons and, above all, the fact that loss of memory is one of its most common features, all contribute to make it difficult, if not impossible, to obtain a reliable history. Furthermore, there are usually many 'red herrings' among the symptoms.

The thought processes which lead to the diagnosis run some-

42

thing like this: the observation of pallor suggests anaemia and therefore a blood count is indicated. The blood count reveals an unexpectedly severe anaemia which is macrocytic in type. This immediately suggests megaloblastic erythropoiesis, the proof of which may be in the peripheral blood and will certainly be in the marrow. Once the presence of megaloblastic erythropoiesis is established, pernicious anaemia becomes the prime suspect. The next step is to test the gastric juice for HCl after histamine stimulation. If HCl is absent, then pernicious anaemia is almost certainly the correct diagnosis. For confirmation, absorption tests or a serum vitamin B_{12} assay may be done.

THE ANAEMIA OF INFECTION

Anaemia is a common occurrence in patients with infections, especially chronic infections. Fortunately, in the vast majority of cases the anaemia is mild and therefore unobtrusive and it is the infection, rather than the anaemia, that occupies our thoughts. But in some cases the anaemia is prominent and demands treatment.

The morphological types

In most cases of anaemia of infection, the anaemia is normochromic normocytic and aregenerative in type. Sometimes, however, it is of the hypochromic microcytic type. There is nothing in the appearance of the red cells to suggest the diagnosis, but when they are hypochromic and microcytic the question of confusion with iron deficiency arises. This will be discussed later.

The pathogenesis of anaemia of infection

In certain infections, notably those due to *Clostridium welchii* and malaria parasites, the anaemia is essentially haemolytic in its pathogenesis. Sometimes, as we have already seen, infection may lead to auto-allergic haemolytic anaemia. In other cases the infection leads to haemorrhage and thus to anaemia.

In the majority of cases, however, the anaemia is due essentially to marrow failure although even in these there may be a haemolytic or a haemorrhagic element.

The common infections which lead to significant anaemia are, bronchiectasis, pulmonary abscess, empyema, subacute bacterial endocarditis, brucellosis, typhoid fever, chronic osteomyelitis and chronic pelvic infections. How exactly these chronic infections lead to anaemia is not completely understood. One view is that the infection disturbs haemoglobin synthesis and that this disturbance involves

43

mainly the globin fraction. Another view is that iron, instead of being incorporated into the haem molecule, is diverted to the stores in the liver and spleen. Yet another view is that infection interferes with the mobilization of iron from the iron stores.

Distinction from iron deficiency anaemia

When hypochromic anaemia occurs in the course of an infection, the problem of distinguishing it from the hypochromic anaemia of chronic haemorrhage and dietary deficiency arises. The clinical features of infection on the one hand, and chronic haemorrhage and dietary deficiency on the other, will be sufficient to make this distinction in most cases. But sometimes there will be doubt, in which event it may be necessary to estimate the serum iron and total iron binding capacity (TIBC). In the iron deficiency cases, the serum iron is reduced but the TIBC is increased; while in hypochromic anaemia due to infection both the serum iron and the TIBC are reduced. This, together with the normal situation is shown graphically in *Figure 2*.

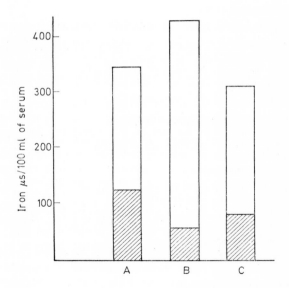

Figure 2. The columns A,B, and C represent TIBC. The shaded areas represent the serum iron content:
A: normal; B: nutritonal iron deficiency or chronic haemorrhage; C: infection

The treatment of the anaemia of infection

If the anaemia is severe, blood transfusion is indicated. If, however, it is mild or moderate, which is more usual, then the treatment is directed to the underlying infection. This, in some cases, may involve operative surgery. With the removal of the infection the haemoglobin concentration will rise without the use of haematinics unless, as not infrequently happens, there is a coincidental deficiency.

The treatment of the anaemia of rheumatoid arthritis requires special mention, not only because it is so common but also because it is so complex. If it is a normochromic normocytic anaemia, which it usually is, then steroid therapy may be followed by an improvement. Transfusion is seldom required. If it is a hypochromic microcytic anaemia, as it often is, then it should be treated as for iron deficiency anaemia, but the usual response is not to be expected until the rheumatoid process has been controlled. Rarely, the anaemia is megaloblastic in type and in these cases vitamin B_{12}, followed if necessary by folic acid, should be tried.

THE ANAEMIA OF RENAL FAILURE

Anaemia is a common accompaniment of renal failure and in many of these cases the haemoglobin level seems to fall as the blood urea level rises. This, however, is not to suggest that the rising urea causes the falling haemoglobin.

Because of the disturbance of fluid balance in these cases, it is quite impossible to assess the degree of anaemia accurately by the ordinary methods, that is, haemoglobin and PCV estimations. However, in most situations, these are all that are available.

Pathogenesis of the anaemia

The anaemia is due mainly to marrow failure; this is shown by radioiron utilization tests. But, in addition, there is a reduced life span of the red cells and sometimes, especially in terminal cases, this is prominent. Haemorrhage often makes a contribution and sometimes a large one. Occasionally, when micro-angiopathy is present, the anaemia is frankly haemolytic in its pathogenesis.

Morphological types of anaemia

In the vast majority of cases the anaemia is normochromic and normocytic in type. Occasionally it is macrocytic or microcytic. Polychromasia is not prominent, but a slightly raised reticulocyte count is often present. Sometimes the full blown picture of micro-angiopathic haemolytic anaemia is seen (*see* Clinical protocol 13).

Treatment

The treatment of the anaemia (and usually the treatment of the cause of the anaemia) is completely unsatisfactory. The only worthwhile remedy is blood transfusion.

Cobaltous chloride has been recommended for the treatment of the anaemia in chronic renal disease. It is, however, questionable if it is of any real value.

It is important to remember that the anaemia in renal disease is probably never as severe as the haemoglobin concentration would suggest. If the renal lesion is treatable, and is successfully treated, the haemoglobin concentration will rise automatically.

Clinical protocol 13. Anaemia in renal failure

A man aged 58 years complained of weakness, cough and swelling of the hands, feet and face. These symptoms had been present for about 2 weeks.

Haemogram

Haemoglobin	8·6 g%	White cell count	5,000/mm^3
		Neutrophils	53%
PCV	26%	Monocytes	3%
		Lymphocytes	44%
MCHC	33%	Eosinophils	0%
		Basophils	0%

The red cells are normochromic and normocytic; they show anisocytosis and some poikilocytosis. The total and differential white cell counts are normal. The platelets are normal in number and appearance.

Comment

The clinical history and the physical findings in this case left little doubt of the diagnosis of renal failure. The haemogram, though of a kind very commonly seen in patients with renal failure, does not contribute to the diagnosis in a positive way. Because the anaemia is normochromic, normocytic and aregenerative in type, it is often said to be due to toxic inhibition of the bone marrow, but no toxin has ever been demonstrated.

Another theory of the pathogenesis of the anaemia in these cases involves the concept of erythropoietin. Erythropoietin is a glycoprotein normally present in the serum. Its concentration increases in response to hypoxia and its function is to stimulate the marrow in regard to red cell production. High levels of erythropoietin have been found in the blood in many kinds of anaemia, but low levels are found in patients with the anaemia of renal failure. Animal experiments suggest that erythropoietin is formed, or at least activated, by the kidneys. It has therefore been suggested that the anaemia in some cases of renal failure is due, in part at least, to failure of the diseased kidneys to form or to activate erythropoietin.

This theory is attractive yet there are some observations which preclude its unqualified acceptance.

ANAEMIA DUE TO DRUGS AND CHEMICALS

Anaemia due to drugs and chemicals requires a literature of its own, which in fact it has. We have already seen how certain drugs may induce haemolytic anaemia by direct toxic action on the red cells, especially those which are deficient in G-6-PD, and how others induce haemolytic anaemia by an auto-allergic mechanism. Later we shall see how a number of drugs, by causing a haemorrhagic disorder, may bring about anaemia by this mechanism. Here, however, we are concerned with drugs which cause anaemia by causing marrow failure.

A list of the more important of these is given on page 90, from which it will be seen that no investigation of an anaemic patient is complete until the question of exposure to drugs (and other noxious chemicals) has been probed. In obscure cases, any drug which the patient may have been taking must be identified and checked for its toxicity.

Morphological types

In typical cases the anaemia is normochromic, normocytic and aregenerative in type. In extreme cases all the cellular elements, red cells, white cells and platelets, are reduced in number. This pancytopenia is characteristic of what is called aplastic anaemia, a name which suggests the state of the bone marrow. In typical cases the bone marrow shows the complete, or almost complete, absence of all nucleated cells except lymphocytes.

Clinical features

The clinical features depend on the anaemia, the neutropenia and the thrombocytopenia. There is therefore pallor and the other variable features of anaemia; infection, usually of the mouth or throat, and

47

purpura. The same syndrome of pancytopenia is found in cases of aleukaemic leukaemia, but in these cases there is usually sternal tenderness and enlargement of lymph glands, liver and spleen, features which are typically absent in aplastic anaemia. The blood picture is nearly always diagnostic and a marrow examination will solve all but the rarest cases (*see* Clinical protocol 14).

Clinical protocol 14. Aplastic anaemia

A woman aged 40 years was suffering from sinusitis, for which her doctor treated her with chloramphenicol. Within a short time a progressive anaemia developed.

Haemogram

Haemoglobin	5·1 g%	White cell count	1,500/mm³
		Neutrophils	2%
PCV	16%	Monocytes	2%
		Lymphocytes	96%
MCHC	32%	Eosinophils	0%
		Basophils	0%

The red cells are normochromic and normocytic; they show no gross pathological change. There is a marked neutropenia. The platelets are greatly reduced in number.

Comment

This haemogram is typical of the kind found in aplastic anaemia, whether the anaemia be due to poisoning or not. In view of the fact that the patient had been taking chloramphenicol, a well known cause of aplastic anaemia, it is reasonable to suppose that that was the cause in this case.

It will be seen that this is more than an anaemia; it is a pancytopenia, red cells, white cells and platelets all being reduced in number. The clinical manifestations are therefore more complex; indeed, those due to the neutropenia (septic sore throat) and the thrombocytopenia (purpura, petechiae, epistaxis) are usually more prominent than those due to the anaemia.

The treatment of this condition consists in discontinuing the offending drug and supporting the patient with transfusions of packed cells. It is usual also to give folic acid and vitamin B_{12} lest these should be deficient. Treatment must be continued until the bone marrow shows signs of recovery. Generally the prognosis is poor, but hope should not be abandoned. The present patient recovered after a few weeks. Sometimes the same blood picture is found in persons who have not been taking drugs and who have not been exposed to noxious chemicals or radiations. Such cases are called primary or idiopathic aplastic anaemia.

THE ANAEMIA OF HYPOTHYROIDISM

Anaemia in hypothyroidism is common but it is not as severe as the pallor in these patients would suggest. It is usually normochromic and normocytic in type, but sometimes it is macrocytic and may therefore be confused with pernicious anaemia. Furthermore, the two conditions, hypothyroidism and pernicious anaemia, occur together more often than can be accounted for by chance. In the macrocytic anaemia of hypothyroidism, however, the macrocytosis is more uniform. This, and other features which can be observed on the blood film will make the distinction in most cases. Sometimes the anaemia is hypochromic and microcytic.

The pathogenesis of the anaemia

The pathogenesis of the anaemia of hypothyroidism is obscure and probably complicated. One view which received considerable support is that the anaemia represents a physiological adjustment of the bone marrow to the diminished need for oxygen which occurs in these patients. However attractive this theory, it leaves certain phenomena unexplained. In particular, it does not explain why only some patients with hypothyroidism develop anaemia, nor does it explain the variations in the morphological types of anaemia that occur.

Treatment

The anaemia responds to treatment by thyroid extract but the response is characteristically slow. This is a point about which the patient should be warned beforehand. Furthermore, the reticulo-cytosis seen in other forms of anaemia after specific treatment does not occur.

If the anaemia is macrocytic in type, then the possibility of a co-existing Addisonian pernicious anaemia must be considered, and, if proven, must be treated accordingly. The treatment of Addisonian pernicious anaemia is discussed on page 53. If, on the other hand, the anaemia is hypochromic and microcytic in type, then the question of iron deficiency anaemia, with all its connotations, must be explored.

5—An Approach to the Investigation of Anaemia

With increasing experience, each doctor develops his own approach to the investigation of anaemia. What follows here is a suggestion for beginners. This approach is based on the method in which anaemia has been presented in the previous pages, but first an important piece of general advice is offered. Find out from a reliable source* the approximate frequency of the various kinds of anaemia which occur in the area where you practice. You may, for example, be in practice in an area where malnutrition, haemoglobinopathy and malaria are common, or in an area where they are rare. This kind of information is usually easily obtained and it is almost indispensable as a background to your thinking.

(1) Approach every case of anaemia in the knowledge that it is due to haemorrhage, excess haemolysis or marrow failure. The history of the case should therefore be taken with a view to answering the three basic questions.

Is there haemorrhage?
Is there excess haemolysis?
Is there marrow failure?

From the accounts previously given, it should be possible to make a shrewd guess at the answers to these questions. One, however, must not expect a clear-cut answer. As has already been seen, more than one of these pathogenetic mechanisms may be operating in a given case, but usually one predominates.

(2) When taking the clinical history, never forget to make a few enquiries about the diet, with a view to assessing if it is reasonably balanced; never forget to enquire about the menstrual history, with a

* The Medical Officer of Health, the local pathologist or an older and more experienced colleague.

view to assessing if there is excessive blood loss; and never forget to enquire about possible drug-taking.

(3) If gastro-intestinal haemorrhage is a possibility, test the stools for occult blood. If the test is positive, a rectal examination and a radiological examination of the gastro-intestinal tract will probably be necessary.

(4) Send a specimen of blood to the laboratory for a blood count. Do not omit to state your suspicion of the pathogenetic mechanism. If you have no suspicions then send the relevant clinical details.

Please remember that from an examination of the blood alone, the pathologist can seldom state the cause of the anaemia. To him, the history of the case is just as important as the specimen.

(5) Where there are absolutely no laboratory facilities, do not forget the therapeutic test. Iron deficiency will respond to iron, folic acid deficiency to folic acid and vitamin B_{12} deficiency to vitamin B_{12}. Do, however, remember the danger of administering folic acid to patients who are deficient in vitamin B_{12} and do not forget to check the results of such specific treatment.

Concerning physical examination, special attention should be paid to the following points.

Conjunctivae	Are they pale or yellow?
Tongue	Is it dry, coated, raw or atrophic?
Lymphatic glands	Are they enlarged?
Sternum	Is there sternal tenderness?
Spleen	Is it enlarged?
Skin	Are there petechiae and ecchymosis or leg ulcers?
Finger nails	Is there koilonychia?
Urine	Is there proteinuria?

Red herrings

Sometimes the clinical features of a case are so bizarre and confusing that 'neurosis' or even 'psychosis' becomes the initial clinical impression. Please be careful. Such cases may be due to Addisonian pernicious anaemia, megaloblastic anaemia from other causes, sickle cell anaemia or a disease which will be considered later, thrombotic thrombocytopenic purpura. A blood examination in these cases will be most rewarding and may save a patient from the psychiatrist.

6—Anaemia: The Principles of Treatment

The first principle in the treatment of any anaemia is to remove the cause of the anaemia. No one has ever discovered what the second principle is.

> Haemorrhages must be stopped.
> Deficiencies must be supplied.
> Infections and infestations must be eliminated.
> Noxious drugs and chemicals must be avoided.

These measures will cater for the vast majority of cases. There will still, however, be a number of cases in which no cause can be found, or, if found, cannot be cured. For these, no general advice can be given; each must be treated as an individual problem.

DRUGS AND PROCEDURES USED IN THE TREATMENT OF ANAEMIA

Blood transfusion

Opinion on the use of blood transfusion in the treatment of anaemia is divided. It is, however, the only method by which anaemia can be cured in a matter of hours; hence it is often used in the treatment of anaemia (of any kind) before surgical operations and before childbirth. It is the only treatment possible in the anaemia of chronic nephritis, aplastic anaemia and severe cases of haemolytic disease of the newborn.

The following points may help as a guide in the use of blood transfusion.

(1) Physicians (as opposed to surgeons) have little need to give whole blood transfusions. Their patients, having sufficient plasma,

need only red cells. A transfusion of packed red cells is therefore the treatment of choice in the vast majority of 'medical' anaemias.

(2) Anaemia following acute haemorrhage must not be confused with shock following acute haemorrhage. The latter is an extreme emergency which must be treated immediately. For this purpose, plasma (or serum or Dextran) should be given immediately. Subsequently the anaemia can be treated by blood transfusion.

(3) As a general rule, blood transfusion should be withheld if the patient's haemoglobin level is 10 g per cent or more. The great exception to this rule is haemolytic disease of the newborn.

(4) Blood transfusion carries a risk, often a risk of death. It should therefore not be undertaken lightly. The hazards of blood transfusion will be considered later; in the meantime it is well to remember that blood is the most potentially dangerous 'drug' which a doctor uses.

Iron

All hypochromic anaemias should be treated with iron notwithstanding the fact that some hypochromic anaemias are not due to iron deficiency. The response, or lack of response, will indicate in the majority of cases if the iron was necessary. This general rule is based on the fact that, after protein deficiency, iron deficiency is the commonest in the world, and it is by far the commonest cause of hypochromic anaemia.

Folic acid

Folic acid has its greatest use in the treatment of nutritional megaloblastic anaemia. It is, however, a dangerous drug and may lead to disastrous results if given in the absence of vitamin B_{12}. If there is doubt as to whether a macrocytic anaemia is due to folic acid or vitamin B_{12} deficiency, and this cannot be resolved, then it is wise to give a protective dose of vitamin B_{12} first.

Vitamin B_{12}

Vitamin B_{12} has its greatest use in the treatment of Addisonian pernicious anaemia. In the absence of signs of malnutrition, all macrocytic anaemias may be treated with vitamin B_{12} in the first instance; however, as pernicious anaemia requires life-long treatment, it is necessary to be reasonably sure of the diagnosis. If a bone marrow examination is to be undertaken, it must be done before vitamin B_{12} (or folic acid) is given to the patient because with this treatment a megaloblastic bone marrow may change to normoblastic in a matter of hours.

Chemotherapy

The anaemias of infection can often be cured by the administration of the appropriate chemotherapeutic agent; often no other treatment is required in these patients. Sometimes, of course, surgery is required to remove the infection. It is important to remember that infection is the commonest cause for failure of specific treatment in folic acid and vitamin B_{12} deficiencies, and it is a very common cause for the failure of iron in nutritional iron deficiency anaemia.

Thyroid extract

The anaemia of hypothyroidism is not usually severe. It responds slowly to the administration of thyroid extract.

ACTH and steroid hormones

ACTH and steroid hormones give excellent results in some cases of acquired haemolytic anaemia, but they are useless in others. Unfortunately there seems to be no reliable means, except trial, of finding out which cases are likely to benefit.

Pyridoxine

Pyridoxine is useful in the treatment of a very rare form of hypochromic anaemia appropriately called 'pyridoxine-responsive anaemia'. When, in the course of treating hypochromic anaemia, it is found that all other methods fail, it would be reasonable to try pyridoxine. But it is important to check for the presence of infection and Mediterranean anaemia in such patients.

Splenectomy

The only absolute indication for splenectomy is hereditary spherocytosis. Certainly not all patients with hereditary spherocytosis require splenectomy; mild cases do not require treatment of any kind. In severe cases, however, it is a most satisfactory procedure as cure is almost certain. Splenectomy is sometimes of value in selected examples of other conditions. If, for example, in Mediterranean anaemia, it can be shown that excessive destruction of red cells is taking place almost exclusively in the spleen, then splenectomy will relieve but, of course, not cure the condition.

7—Myeloproliferative Diseases

The prefix '*myelo*' comes from the Greek word *myelos* meaning marrow. The myeloproliferative diseases therefore consist of a group of disorders which have in common proliferation of marrow cells. This concept of myeloproliferative disease is ill-defined, but nevertheless useful. It does not include the myeloproliferation which occurs in folic acid, vitamin B_{12} and iron deficiency, nor does it include the proliferation of cells which occurs in haemorrhage, infections and secondary polycythaemia. It may, however, be used to denote a group which includes the following: polycythaemia vera, leukaemia, myelofibrosis, erythroleukaemia of Di Guglielmo, myelomatosis and essential thrombocythaemia.

CYTOGENESIS

No reasonable view of these myeloproliferative diseases is possible except through that approach which takes into consideration the cytogenesis of the blood and allied cells. Unfortunately, this cytogenesis is not fully known, but the following is a reasonable working account of it.

The primitive mesenchymal cell of Maximow persists in adult life, and is found in association with the cells of the reticulo-endothelial system. It is the ancestor of all the cells of mesodermal tissue, of which blood is an example. From it therefore are derived red cells, white cells, platelets, plasma cells, fibrocytes and osteocytes. It is, in short, a multipotential cell.

As a result of stimulation it may give rise to one or more of these various cell types; thus a line of erythroid cells, myeloid cells and fibrocytes may develop more or less simultaneously. But one or other of these cell types usually predominates, giving rise to a characteristic

55

microscopic appearance. Often, after a period of domination, this one cell type gives way and another type dominates the picture. Thus, in polycythaemia vera, red cells predominate but there is nearly always an increase in white cells and platelets also. Towards the end of the disease it is not infrequent for the white cells to become dominant and so, what began as polycythaemia vera, ends up as chronic myeloid leukaemia. Similarly, in myelofibrosis, fibrous tissue predominates in the bone marrow, but usually white cells and platelets are increased as well, and not infrequently frank leukaemia supervenes. Acute erythroleukaemia may end as leukaemia or vice versa, and a leuco-erythroblastic reaction sometimes occurs in myelomatosis. Thus it is stressed that disease processes are not to be considered analogous to plant species as Sydenham and Cohnheim would have us believe.

Clinico-pathological features

The symptoms and signs of the myeloproliferative diseases vary greatly depending on which cell type is involved. In myelofibrosis and chronic myeloid leukaemia, massive enlargement of the spleen, and the symptoms and signs which stem from this enlargement are the most conspicuous clinical features. In polycythaemia vera, on the other hand, enlargement of the spleen occurs in little more than 50 per cent of patients and ruddy cyanosis is the most constant clinical feature. In acute leukaemia, anaemia, neutropenia and thrombocytopenia are responsible for the main clinical manifestations, while in chronic lymphatic leukaemia, splenomegaly and generalized enlargement of the lymphatic glands form the characteristic clinical picture. In myelomatosis, bone pain (often low back pain) is the most common presenting symptom, and splenomegaly occurs in only about 10 per cent of cases.

It is therefore clear that little can be said about the group as a whole which would be applicable to each of its members. It is for this reason that the most important members of the group must now be considered individually.

MYELOFIBROSIS

Myelofibrosis is characterized histologically by a proliferation of fibrous tissue in the bone marrow. This characterization, however, is not visible to the clinician. Coincidentally, myeloid metaplasia occurs in the liver and spleen resulting in an enlargement of these organs which may be massive. This is the most conspicuous clinical feature of the disease. These basic pathological changes cause secondary changes in the circulating blood which are described as leuco-erythroblastic anaemia, or myelophthisic anaemia.

The symptoms are vague or misleading, and it is usually not until the enlarged spleen is discovered that the various complaints begin to arrange themselves into a possible diagnosis. In most cases, however, it is the enlargement of the spleen, or the symptoms which stem from the enlargement, which call attention to the disease in the first place. Among the symptoms attributable to splenomegaly are swelling of the abdomen, a feeling of fullness or weight in the abdomen and a dragging pain in the splenic area. Enlargement of the liver, though common, is not as common nor as prominent as enlargement of the spleen. The combined enlargements of the liver and the spleen cause an increase in the intra-abdominal pressure and this causes partial occlusion of the great veins with resulting oedema of the lower limbs. A bleeding tendency is not uncommon at some stage of the disease; it may take the form of petechiae or ecchymosis.

Blood picture

The blood picture is discussed on page 19.

Diagnosis

It is not possible to recognize myelofibrosis at the bedside, but the discovery of a massively enlarged spleen must suggest both myelo-fibrosis and chronic myeloid leukaemia. The blood picture, if characteristic, will suggest myelofibrosis; it will certainly exclude chronic myeloid leukaemia. Radiological examination of the bones may help, but the final confirmation is by bone marrow examination and in this connection it is stressed that simple aspiration is not sufficient; one must have recourse to surgical biopsy.

Treatment

There is no satisfactory treatment. Generally speaking, attempts should be made to treat that aspect of the disease which is causing the greatest concern. Busulphan (Myleran) has been used to reduce the size of the spleen.

Clinical protocol 15.   Myelofibrosis

A girl aged 17 years was admitted to hospital with a variety of chronic complaints which included weakness, dyspnoea, chest pain, abdominal discomfort and swelling of the feet. On exam-ination, the patient was found to have marked enlargement of the liver, massive enlargement of the spleen and bilateral oedema of the feet.

Haemogram

Haemoglobin	8·5 g%	White cell count	18,000/mm³
		Neutrophils	55%
PCV	28%	Monocytes	0%
		Lymphocytes	6%
MCHC	34%	Eosinophils	1%
		Basophils	0%
		Metamyelocytes	6%
		Myelocytes	12%
		Promyelocytes	9%
		Myeloblasts	11%

The red cells are normochromic and normocytic; they show anisocytosis, poikilocytosis, increased diffuse polychromasia and nucleated forms. There is a leucocytosis with a marked shift to the left. Platelets are increased in number (865,000/mm³) and occasional giant forms were seen.

Comment

Bone marrow aspiration was attempted, and after one or two failures a reasonably satisfactory specimen was obtained. It showed a slightly hypocellular marrow with a shift to the left of the erythroid and myeloid cells. Later, a portion of bone was resected for histological examination. This showed fibrosis of the marrow cavity, which explained the difficulty in obtaining a marrow specimen by aspiration, and which permitted a diagnosis of myelofibrosis. After some months, the total white cell count had risen to 400,000/mm³. At this stage it was reasonable to regard the case as chronic myeloid leukaemia.

This is an example of a myeloproliferative disease which began as myelofibrosis and ended as chronic myeloid leukaemia. The transition from myelofibrosis to leukaemia is a gradual process and any attempt to define the precise time must be purely arbitrary.

Although it was strongly suspected by the clinical features and the haemogram, even the failed marrow aspiration was a clue, the final proof depended on a histological examination of the bone marrow.

CHRONIC MYELOID LEUKAEMIA

Chronic myeloid leukaemia is slow in its onset and in its course, and it is invariably fatal. It is essentially a disease of middle age, the vast majority of cases occurring between 30 and 60 years of age.

The presenting symptoms are usually vague and consist of tiredness, weakness, loss of weight and abdominal discomfort. Often there are many other symptoms, not directly related to the basic myeloproliferative process, such as cough, breathlessness and swelling of the feet. In fact there may be so many complaints that it is difficult to focus attention on any one of them.

The most significant, and usually the most prominent, complaint is of abdominal discomfort. This is due to a massive enlargement of the spleen and may be described as a 'dragging' pain (due to the weight of the spleen) or a more acute pain (due to infarction or perisplenitis). The most striking feature on physical examination is the enlarged spleen. It is the largest which the average doctor is likely to encounter in his career. It often reaches into the pelvis and on occasions it may be so large as to simulate an advanced pregnancy.

Blood picture

A normochromic normocytic regenerative anaemia is nearly always present, but the distinctive feature is a marked leucocytosis with a shift to the left. A similar picture is occasionally found in other conditions such as tuberculosis and disseminated carcinoma. Such leukaemoid blood pictures sometimes cause difficulty but, if viewed in the light of the clinical features, the difficulties usually fade. The presence of large numbers of basophils and the reduction of the enzyme alkaline phosphatase in the granulocytes are sometimes useful distinguishing features between leukaemia, when they are expected, and leukaemoid reactions when they are not.

Diagnosis

Because of the great variety and indefinite nature of the symptoms of which the patient may complain, it might be thought that chronic myeloid leukaemia is a difficult disease to recognize; in fact it is not. The key to the diagnosis is in the recognition of the enlarged spleen. Once this has been recognized, the correct diagnosis must inevitably follow. The blood picture will confirm the diagnosis in 99 per cent of cases. I have never known a bone marrow examination to be necessary.

Treatment

Although some doctors recommend radiotherapy (usually radiotherapists), most use drug treatment. The drug of choice is Busulphan or, as it is more commonly known, Myleran. The usual dose is 4 mg daily.

During the first month of treatment there is a fairly rapid, but

59

nevertheless variable, fall in the total white cell count. When it reaches about 10,000 to 12,000/mm³, the treatment may be discontinued for a period. Thereafter it may be resumed when indicated. With the fall in the white cell count there is a rise in the haemoglobin concentration and the patient feels much better.

Later in the course of the disease blood transfusion may be required.

Treatment does not cure the disease; it is questionable if it even prolongs life, but it does make the patient feel better. That is all that can be done at the present time.

Prognosis

Some patients die within 12 months, others may survive for 12 years. At the beginning it is not possible to say which patients are likely to survive and hence it is quite impossible to prognosticate.

Chronic myeloid leukaemia sometimes ends as acute leukaemia, but more often death is due to haemorrhage or an intercurrent infection.

Clinical protocol 16.   Chronic myeloid leukaemia

A man aged 59 years was admitted to hospital because of pain and swelling of the feet, pain in the chest on coughing and abdominal pain. These symptoms had been present for an indefinite period of time but probably in the region of 2 months. On examination the main clinical findings were bilateral oedema of the feet, a greatly enlarged spleen and a slightly enlarged liver. There was no lymph glandular enlargement and no sternal tenderness.

Haemogram

Haemoglobin	7·9 g%	White cell count	310,000/mm³
		Neutrophils	58%
PCV	25%	Monocytes	5%
		Lymphocytes	2%
MCHC	32%	Eosinophils	5%
		Basophils	8%
		Metamyelocytes	6%
		Myelocytes	8%
		Promyelocytes	3%
		Myeloblasts	5%

The red cells are normochromic and normocytic; they show anisocytosis, poikilocytosis, increased diffuse polychromasia and nucleated forms. There is a marked leucocytosis with a marked shift to the left. Platelets are greatly increased in number (935,000/mm³).

Comment

Here is another example of a myeloproliferative disease. This time the diagnosis was chronic myeloid leukaemia. It will be noted that the white cells and platelets are in the ascendency. Notice also the similarities in both the clinical features and blood findings between this and the previous case. Massive spleens must always suggest myelofibrosis and chronic myeloid leukaemia.

This blood picture could hardly be due to anything else but chronic myeloid leukaemia. Occasionally, however, a similar blood picture is encountered in non-leukaemia patients; such are called leukaemoid reactions. One useful way of distinguishing between the leukaemic and the leukaemoid pictures is to consider the basophils. In chronic myeloid leukaemia they are usually present in abundance, while in the leukaemoid picture they are few or absent.

POLYCYTHAEMIA VERA

Polycythaemia vera is slow in its onset and usually slow in its course. The presenting symptoms are vague and varied: headache, breathlessness, dizziness, abdominal discomfort, chest pain, visual disturbances, pruritus and epistaxis are fairly common complaints, but sometimes there is no complaint whatsoever. One of my patients presented with gangrene of a toe but with no other clinical manifestation of polycythaemia. The case was exposed when a routine haemoglobin estimation was done.

In some patients there is a characteristic facies, usually described as a ruddy cyanosis. When present in its fully developed form it enables the disease to be recognized at a glance, but it is present in only about 50 per cent of patients. Enlargement of the spleen is commonly found and sometimes it is a marked enlargement. Enlargement of the liver is less common.

Blood picture

There is an increase in the haemoglobin concentration and the PCV. Haemoglobin values of more than 20 g per cent are quite common. The PCV is raised proportionately; hence the MCHC is normal. Occasionally, as a result of bleeding, the MCHC is low. The red cells in uncomplicated cases are normochromic and normocytic.

They show slight anisocytosis and slightly increased diffuse poly-chromasia. A few normoblasts and an occasional red cell showing punctate basophilia are often seen. If there has been chronic haemor-rhage, the red cells may be hypochromic and microcytic.

There is often, but not always, a neutrophilia with a shift to the left. The total white cell count, however, is usually not markedly in-creased; counts of about 15,000/mm^3 are common but they may be well in excess of this.

The blood platelets are often increased in number, values of over a million are not infrequent.

Diagnosis

In those 50 per cent of patients who present the characteristic facies, polycythaemia vera is immediately recognized. In the other 50 per cent, diagnosis on clinical grounds is impossible. There may, however, be some feature in the clinical picture which will demand a blood count and this will immediately expose the polycythaemia. Often it is brought to light by a routine haemoglobin estimation.

As already said, the blood count will immediately show that the patient has polycythaemia; it then remains to prove that it is primary and not secondary polycythaemia. The neutrophilia and the thrombo-cytosis, if present, will be strong evidence in favour of the primary condition but it is advisable to exclude as far as possible all the causes of secondary polycythaemia. These include heart disease, lung disease, methaemoglobinaemia, sulphaemoglobinaemia and those lesions of the brain, pituitary, kidney, liver and elsewhere which are rarely associated with polycythaemia. The extent of the investiga-tions required will depend on the circumstances that obtain in the individual patient.

Treatment

Two forms of treatment are in common use, venesection and ^{32}P. Each has its advocates and some alternate between one and the other. No schedule of treatment can be laid down, as the disease process varies greatly from one patient to another. Because of the essentially chronic nature of the disease, patients come to know when they should be bled or when they should have more ^{32}P.

Radiotherapy has been used with success but most doctors prefer the other methods.

Prognosis

The disease is incurable but many patients survive for 10–15 years, and during this time they are reasonably comfortable. Thrombosis and haemorrhage are the main complications and they may occur at any time during the course of the disease. They are the commonest cause of death. Sometimes the disease ends as chronic myeloid leukaemia, less commonly it ends as acute leukaemia.

Clinical protocol 17. Polycythaemia vera

A man aged 54 years was admitted to hospital complaining of severe headache, breathlessness and dizziness. These symptoms had been present for about 12 months. In more recent months he complained, in addition, of pruritus. On clinical examination, the main points noted were a ruddy complexion, a raised blood pressure and an enlarged spleen. Several blood counts were done of which the following is typical.

Haemogram

Haemoglobin	21 g%	White cell count	18,000/mm^3
		Neutrophils	73%
PCV	60%	Monocytes	8%
		Lymphocytes	19%
MCHC	35%	Eosinophils	0%
		Basophils	0%

The red cells are normochromic and normocytic. They show slight anisocytosis and slightly increased diffuse polychromasia. There is a neutrophilia with a slight shift to the left. Platelets are increased in number.

Comment

This is yet another example of a myeloproliferative disease. In this case the diagnosis is primary polycythaemia, otherwise known as polycythaemia vera. Secondary polycythaemia is not included among the myeloproliferative diseases; it is distinguished from the primary type, in typical cases, by the absence of the changes in the white cells and platelets.

Primary polycythaemia may prove fatal from haemorrhage or thrombosis, but sometimes as the disease progresses the haemoglobin concentration and the PCV fall, the pathological changes in the white cells become more prominent and thus the disease passes gradually into chronic myeloid leukaemia.

Occasionally, a rather disconcerting feature occurs in the red cells of patients with polycythaemia vera. Instead of being normochromic they become hypochromic. This is usually due to iron deficiency resulting from the therapeutic bleeding.

ACUTE LEUKAEMIA

Acute leukaemia is a fatal condition characterized by excessive proliferation of white cells. Usually these cells appear in the peripheral blood, giving rise to a marked leucocytosis. The word leukaemia means 'white blood'. This is a misnomer because the blood is never white; furthermore, the total white cell count is sometimes normal or even below normal. Such cases are called aleukaemic leukaemia and in them the excessive proliferation can be demonstrated in the bone marrow.

Three main types of acute leukaemia are recognized depending on the particular cell type involved in the proliferative process.

(1) Acute myeloblastic leukaemia.
(2) Acute lymphoblastic leukaemia.
(3) Acute monoblastic leukaemia.

The myeloblast, lymphoblast and monoblast are so alike that it is often difficult or impossible to distinguish them. For this reason the non-committal term 'acute blast cell leukaemia' is often used. Acute leukaemia occurs most commonly in childhood and is usually of the lymphoblastic type.

Blood picture

Anaemia is an almost constant concomitant of acute leukaemia. It is normochromic, normocytic and regenerative in type. Sometimes it is mild but if left untreated it always becomes severe. It is probably haemolytic in its pathogenesis but haemorrhage and marrow failure no doubt contribute.

The white cell count is usually high but it may be normal or low (aleukaemic leukaemia). It may vary from 500 to 100,000/mm³. The most significant finding is the presence of primitive cells, lymphoblasts, myeloblasts or monoblasts. These cells constitute up to 95 per cent of the total count. Because of this, a neutropenia is commonly present and this leads to sepsis.

Thrombocytopenia occurs in some 90 per cent of cases of acute leukaemia and it is responsible for the bleeding tendency which is often among the most prominent early signs.

Clinical picture

The clinical picture of acute leukaemia varies greatly from patient to patient. In a typical case there is pyrexia and this often suggests an acute infection. Enlargement of the spleen, liver and lymphatic glands are common but most important of all is sternal tenderness. The other clinical features can be related to the major blood changes as follows:

(1) Anaemia leads to pallor, loss of energy and prostration.

(2) Neutropenia leads to sepsis, especially oral sepsis.

(3) Thrombocytopenia leads to epistaxis, purpura and petechiae.

Diagnosis

Because of its variable clinical picture, the disease is often mis-diagnosed or not diagnosed at the bedside. One clinical sign which stands out above all others and unfortunately is often neglected is sternal tenderness. The importance of this sign cannot be over-stressed, indeed the young doctor would be well advised to test for it in all his patients. Using the tips of the fingers or thumb, the sternum should be firmly pressed along its entire length from the manubrium to the xiphoid process. Experience will show the amount of pressure to apply but it is well to apply light pressure at first. When this is done, the patient with acute leukaemia will often wince or cry out with pain. This sign is not completely specific for acute leukaemia, but it is so commonly present that it is one of the most valuable signs in the whole of clinical medicine.

A blood count will confirm the diagnosis in the vast majority of cases but occasionally, in the aleukaemic phase, it may be necessary to do a bone marrow examination.

Treatment

In its natural course, acute leukaemia, although subject to re-missions, is fatal within 1–2 years and often within 6 months. With the remedies now available it is possible not only to induce much longer remissions and thus prolong life for a number of years, but also to make life much more comfortable for the patient.

For acute lymphoblastic leukaemia, prednisone and mercapto-purine are the most popular drugs at the present time. Other drugs which may be tried in refractory cases are methotrexate, cyclophosphamide and vincristine.

More recently, asparaginase, an enzyme which splits asparagine* has become established as an effective remedy for bringing about remissions in these patients and more recently still, very good results have been reported by McElwain and Hardisty using a combination of asparaginase and cytosine arabinoside. An entirely different

---

* Asparagine is not on the official list of essential amino acids because it can be synthetized by normal mammalian tissues. Certain tumours, however, notably lymphoblastic leukaemia and reticulum cell sarcoma, lack this ability. For such growths, therefore, asparagine is an essential amino acid.

approach is that of Mathe. He has had remarkable results using immunological methods in conjunction with chemotherapy.

Less hope can be offered for acute myeloblastic and acute mono-blastic leukaemia. Mercaptopurine is not as effective in these as it is in acute lymphoblastic leukaemia but a new drug, daunorubicin, shows promise.

Apart from the specific treatment mentioned above, it is usually necessary to support patients sooner or later with blood transfusion. In this matter, packed cells should be used rather than whole blood.

Clinical protocol 18.   Acute leukaemia

A girl aged 12 years was brought to hospital because of breath-lessness on exertion and pain in the left hypochondrium. On examination she was found to have marked pallor of her mucous membranes, enlargement of the cervical and submandi-bular lymphatic glands, enlargement of the spleen and marked sternal tenderness. Nothing else of significance was noted.

Haemogram

Haemoglobin	3·0 g%	White cell count	73,000/mm^3
		Neutrophils	4%
PCV	9%	Monocytes	0%
		Lymphocytes	2%
MCHC	33%	Eosinophils	0%
		Basophils	0%
		Blast cells	94%

The red cells are normochromic and normocytic. They show anisocytosis, some poikilocytosis and increased diffuse poly-chromasia. Two normoblasts were seen while counting 100 white cells in the differential white cell count. The white cells show a marked shift to the left. The platelets are greatly reduced in number (14,000/mm^3).

Comment

The clinical history in this case is as typical as one is likely to encounter. The most suggestive features are the enlargement of the spleen and lymphatic glands and the sternal tenderness. Together, these make the bedside diagnosis of acute leukaemia almost certain. Although mentioned last here, sternal tenderness is a particularly suggestive feature and it is often overlooked. It should be sought in all cases; it is a little test which lends charm to the investigation.

If there was any doubt about the diagnosis of acute leukaemia, it is completely dispelled by the haemogram which will permit of no other. A bone marrow examination is therefore unnecessary in this case.

That there are no haemorrhagic manifestations such as ecchymosis, petechiae and epistaxis is rather remarkable. It shows, however, that bleeding tendencies are dependent not only on platelet numbers but on other factors as well. These will be discussed later.

CHRONIC LYMPHATIC LEUKAEMIA

Chronic lymphatic leukaemia is even slower in its onset and course than chronic myeloid leukaemia and its maximum incidence is in an older age group. Because of this, it is not uncommon to discover the condition in a person over 70 years of age who seeks medical advice for some trivial complaint.

The presenting symptoms are vague and often irrelevant, but generalized enlargement of the lymphatic glands is usually prominent and dominates the clinical picture. The enlargement is most noticeable in the superficial cervical glands, but deep glands are involved also and these may give rise to a variety of clinical effects in both the thorax and abdomen. The spleen is always enlarged but the massive enlargement of chronic myeloid leukaemia is not seen. A variety of skin lesions may occur some of which are due to leukaemic infiltration of the skin, others are due to infection. Purpura sometimes occurs towards the end.

Blood picture

A normochromic normocytic regenerative anaemia nearly always occurs, but in the early stages it may be absent. Often it is auto-allergic in origin and the auto-antibodies may give rise to difficulty during transfusion. The most characteristic feature of the blood picture, however, is a marked leucocytosis with so-called mature lymphocytes constituting up to 99 per cent of the white cells. Total white cell counts of from 100,000 to 200,000/mm^3 are quite common. The platelets are usually normal but towards the end thrombocytopenia is common.

Diagnosis

The symptoms are vague and therefore not helpful in diagnosis. Fortunately the signs are most helpful. Generalized, enlarged, discrete, painless lymphatic glands, together with an enlargement of the spleen in a patient of middle age or beyond, is highly suggestive of chronic lymphatic leukaemia. If the young doctor resolves always to do a blood count whenever he encounters enlarged lymphatic glands or an enlarged spleen, he will probably never miss a case of this condition. Bone marrow examination or lymphatic gland biopsy is seldom, if ever, necessary.

Treatment

The first point to decide is whether or not treatment is really required. The disease is so chronic and so slow that many patients do not require treatment when the condition is first discovered. If it is decided that treatment is required, it should be directed towards that aspect of the disease which is demanding attention.

Chlorambucil is the drug of choice but its use, as with all such chemotherapeutic agents, must be controlled with blood counts. The total white cell count should not be allowed to go below about 15,000/mm^3 and any significant drop in the platelet count is the signal to discontinue treatment. Should an accompanying haemolytic anaemia or thrombocytopenia be causing discomfort, then steroid hormones may be used.

Immunological complications

Sometimes chronic lymphatic leukaemia is complicated by agammaglobulinaemia in which event the expected iso-antibodies are absent. This leads to anomalous results during blood grouping. Thus, a blood specimen may appear as group A when the cells are tested, but as group AB when the serum is tested. Such results are always disconcerting and lead to delays in the blood bank. More often, chronic lymphatic leukaemia, in common with other lymphomas such as Hodgkin's disease, is complicated by auto-allergic haemolytic anaemia in which event auto-antibodies appear in the blood. These may cause difficulties in both grouping and cross-matching.

All these difficulties fade or even disappear if the blood bank is advised of the diagnosis when the blood is ordered for the patient. If this simple precaution is taken, much unnecessary work, with its attendant delays, is avoided.

Prognosis

In general, the prognosis is better than in chronic myeloid leukaemia. Many patients live comfortably for 10–20 years, only to die of perhaps an entirely unrelated condition. Other patients, however, deteriorate much more rapidly and may die within 1 or 2 years of diagnosis. Death is usually due to an intercurrent infection or haemorrhage.

Clinical protocol 19.   Chronic lymphatic leukaemia

A woman aged 39 years was admitted to hospital because of an obvious exfoliative dermatitis. This had been present for about 3 years. On further examination she was found to have an enlarged spleen and enlarged cervical and axillary lymphatic glands. The initial diagnosis was Hodgkin's disease.

Haemogram

Haemoglobin	10·3 g%	White cell count	258,000/mm³
		Neutrophils	9%
PCV	33%	Monocytes	1%
		Lymphocytes	89%
MCHC	32%	Eosinophils	1%
		Basophils	0%

The red cells are normochromic and normocytic; they show anisocytosis, increased diffuse polychromasia and occasional nucleated forms. In addition, spherocytes were seen. There is a marked leucocytosis which is essentially a lymphocytosis. The platelets are reduced in number.

Comment

Except in so far as the patient is unusually young, the clinical features in this case are fairly typical of chronic lymphatic leukaemia. They do, however, also suggest Hodgkin's disease which was the original clinical diagnosis. The haemogram resolved the problem.

The blood picture in chronic lymphatic leukaemia contrasts markedly with that in chronic myeloid leukaemia. Nowhere do we see the great variety in cellular form and maturity; the vast majority of the white cells seem to be ordinary mature lymphocytes. Among the red cells, spherocytes are not uncommon in patients with chronic lymphatic leukaemia and other malignant lymphomas; they signify a concomitant haemolytic anaemia of the auto-allergic type. Thrombocytopenia is not infrequent in the late stages of this disease, and it may lead to haemorrhagic phenomena. It, too, is probably due to the auto-allergic process.

MYELOMATOSIS

In myelomatosis there is malignant proliferation of plasma cells in the bone marrow and elsewhere. If there is only one focus of proliferation the condition is referred to as solitary myeloma, but if there are more than one it is called multiple myeloma. The vast majority of patients are over the age of 50 years, and it is about twice as common in males as in females.

The commonest symptom is bone pain which is usually situated in the lumbar region. The other clinical features are much less common and consist of renal failure and a bleeding tendency such as epistaxis, purpura, or prolonged bleeding after a tooth extraction. At a later stage, spontaneous fractures and collapse of the vertebrae may occur which of course lead to secondary effects.

One feature more than any other sets myelomatosis apart from the other myeloproliferative diseases; the malignant plasma cells produce an abnormal protein in large amounts. This paraprotein, as it is often called, is usually related to immunoglobulin G, but it may be related to IgA, IgM, or IgD. The paraprotein may be present in such large amounts that it causes a marked increase in the viscosity of the blood leading to mental symptoms, heart failure and blindness. The bleeding tendency also is probably due to the hyperviscosity. The excess protein in the blood leads to two important and related effects: increased rouleaux formation and a raised blood sedimentation rate.

Blood picture

In the majority of cases there is a normochromic normocytic anaemia. Signs of regeneration may or may not be present, but increased rouleaux formation is nearly always present, and some-times it is so pronounced that it is impossible to make a satisfactory blood film. The white cells vary; they may be increased, normal or decreased. Usually there is nothing of note in the differential count, but occasionally plasma cells are seen.

The platelet count is usually normal but it may be reduced. The sedimentation rate is nearly always greatly increased.

Diagnosis

Headache and backache are two common presenting symptoms of myelomatosis. They are also among the most common symptoms encountered in general practice and the most difficult to evaluate in the whole of clinical medicine. Hence myelomatosis is seldom, if ever, diagnosed at the bedside.

Examination of the blood hardly ever gives definite proof but it often gives two highly suggestive clues: an unexpectedly high blood sedimentation rate and excessive rouleaux formation on the blood film. Once the condition is suggested, a number of confirmatory tests can be done. The more important of these are a radiological examination of the skeleton, electrophoresis or immunoelectrophoresis of the serum proteins, and a microscopic examination of the bone

MYELOMATOSIS

marrow. The ultimate diagnosis is usually based on the evidence of one or more of these procedures.

Treatment

Cyclophosphamide and melphalan (Alkeran) are the drugs of choice. Various treatment schedules have been recommended and sometimes prednisolone has been incorporated with the melphalan regimen. Drug treatment should be controlled with frequent blood counts. Blood transfusions may be required for the anaemia, and if the hyperviscosity syndrome is present then plasmaphaeresis should be undertaken.

Because of the low level of normal IgG, the renal lesions and the drug treatment already recommended, patients with myelomatosis are particularly prone to infections. Such infections demand prompt treatment whenever they arise and, as far as possible, they should be prevented.

Bone pain may be relieved by deep radiotherapy, but if this is not available one must resort to pethedine or morphine. Little or nothing can be done for the renal failure.

Prognosis

The disease is invariably fatal. Most patients are dead within a year; a few survive for 2 years and occasionally longer. The prognosis depends on the incidence of the complications, especially renal failure, infection and haemorrhage. The blood urea is a useful prognostic guide; values of 100 mg/100 ml or more indicate an extremely poor outlook.

Clinical protocol 20.   Myelomatosis

A man aged 70 years was admitted to hospital because of a productive cough, low back pain which had been present for about 3 months and a slight limp which he had developed recently. There was no enlargement of the liver, spleen or lymphatic glands and there was no sternal tenderness.

Haemogram

Haemoglobin	8·2 g%	White cell count	13,000/mm^3
		Neutrophils	70%
PCV	27%	Monocytes	4%
		Lymphocytes	24%
MCHC	30%	Eosinophils	1%
		Basophils	0%
		Plasma cells	1%

71

The red cells are normochromic and normocytic; they show anisocytosis and slightly increased diffuse polychromasia. Rouleaux formation is prominent. There is a slight neutrophilia. The platelets are normal in number and appearance.

Comment

There is no such thing as a typical history or a typical blood picture of myelomatosis. Concerning the clinical features, I make it a rough general rule not to consider the diagnosis in patients under 50 years of age and not to consider it unless there is bone pain.* I make it a rule to consider it strongly whenever I see an unexpectedly high blood sedimentation rate or excessive rouleaux formation on the blood film. Each of these rules have led me astray on occasions, but I still believe that they are useful guides.

The most significant feature in this haemogram is the increased rouleaux formation and it was this that suggested the diagnosis in the first place. The occasional plasma cell has no real significance at all. They are not infrequently seen in the blood of patients who certainly have not got myelomatosis. The diagnosis in this patient was confirmed by finding masses of abnormal plasma cells in the bone marrow.

Although this case illustrates many of the features of myelomatosis, there was one rather strange anomaly, the blood sedimentation rate was 2 mm (Wintrobe).

* As I write these lines, my secretary tells me that a friend of hers died of myelomatosis at 28 years of age.

8—Haemorrhagic Diseases

The haemorrhagic diseases include a number of conditions which are characterized by the occurrence of haemorrhage for little or no apparent reason. It is the trivial nature of the precipitating cause of the haemorrhage which is the hall-mark of these diseases. Thus, a person who bleeds from the nose spontaneously has a haemorrhagic disease, but a person who bleeds from the nose as a result of a blow does not have a haemorrhagic disease.

In haemorrhagic diseases the bleeding is nearly always from multiple sites. This is another helpful distinguishing feature, and it underlines the fact that these are general and not local diseases. Finally, as these diseases are often chronic and often inherited, there is nearly always a history of previous bleeding episodes and sometimes there is a family history of the same kind of bleeding.

The main points therefore in recognizing a haemorrhagic disease are as follows.

(1) Haemorrhage for little or no apparent reason.
(2) Prolonged haemorrhage for trivial reasons.
(3) Haemorrhage from multiple sites.
(4) History of previous episodes of haemorrhage.
(5) Sometimes a family history of similar haemorrhages.

It is stressed that the recognition of a haemorrhagic disease is a task for the bedside, but the diagnosis of the particular type of haemorrhagic disease is a task for the laboratory.

The haemostatic mechanism

Before proceeding further, a short review of the haemostatic mechanism is necessary.

If, as a result of injury, blood escapes from a blood vessel, a series of events take place which have as their end the stoppage of the haemorrhage. These events constitute the haemostatic mechanism and, although they are inter-related, they are conveniently considered under three separate headings: vascular contraction, platelet agglutination, and clotting.

Vascular contraction

In the smallest vessels, reflex contraction is sufficient to obliterate the lumen and thus stop the haemorrhage. In larger vessels, arteries, because they contain much more muscle tissue than veins, can contract more efficiently. This advantage, however, is partly offset by the greater pressure of the blood in the arteries. Nevertheless, haemorrhage from even medium sized arteries, such as the brachial and femoral, is often checked by this mechanism.

Platelet agglutination

Platelets, by agglutinating and undergoing the phenomenon known as viscous metamorphosis, provide a plug which seals the rent in injured blood vessels. In addition, by liberating noradrenaline and 5-hydroxytryptamine, they contribute to the vascular contraction. Finally, by reacting with other plasma constituents, platelets can initiate clotting.

Clotting

Clotting is a complicated process yet the essential facts for our purpose are not difficult to grasp. The process is divided into 3 phases.

Phase 1. Thromboplastin generation.
Phase 2. The conversion of prothrombin to thrombin.
Phase 3. The conversion of fibrinogen to fibrin.

Defects may occur in any one ot these phases and they are usually due to a deficiency of one or more of the factors required for clotting. Thus haemophilia is a defect of phase 1, hypoprothrombinaemia is a defect of phase 2 and fibrinogenopenia is a defect of phase 3. Rarely is a clotting defect due to the presence of a circulating anticoagulant.

The clotting factors

At the present time 12 different clotting factors are known. In 1957, an international committee recommended that Roman numerals be used to designate these various factors but this recommendation has been largely ignored in both life and literature. Thus, calcium is always called calcium and never factor IV. Table 2 lists the clotting factors together with their most commonly used alternative names.

TABLE 2
Clotting Factors and their Synonyms

Factor I	Fibrinogen
Factor II	Prothrombin
Factor III	Thromboplastin
Factor IV	Calcium
Factor V	Labile factor
Factor VI	(none)*
Factor VII	Stable factor
Factor VIII	Antihaemophilic factor (AHF)
Factor IX	Christmas factor
Factor X	Stuart–Prower factor
Factor XI	Plasma thromboplastin antecedent (PTA)
Factor XII	Hageman factor
Factor XIII	Fibrin stabilizing factor

* It will be noted that there is no factor VI. This numeral was originally used to designate what was thought to be an active form of Factor V.

The pathogenesis of the haemorrhagic diseases

We may presume that in the ordinary course of living we are continually breaching the walls of small blood vessels. That haemorrhage does not occur as often as the walls are breached is due to the immediate action of the haemostatic mechanism. If, however, one or more of the elements of this mechanism is defective, then haemorrhage of greater or lesser degree is likely to occur.

However, it must be remembered that haemostasis is a complex mechanism and that therefore there is no direct correlation between the observable defect and the degree of haemorrhage. Thus, while bleeding may be expected when the platelet count falls to about 50,000/mm³, it is not uncommon to find patients with platelet counts well below this level who have no evidence of bleeding. Similarly, the antihaemophilic factor content cannot be directly related to the degree of bleeding suffered by a haemophilic. Table 3 gives a variety of haemorrhagic diseases together with the important pathogenetic factor in each.

The classification of the haemorrhagic diseases

For clinical purposes the haemorrhagic diseases are conveniently divided into two groups.

(1) The clotting diseases (of which haemophilia is the prototype).

(2) The purpuras (of which Werlhof's disease is the prototype).

The distinction between the two can often be made at the bedside. The key manifestations of a clotting disease are haemarthrosis and haematomas, while those of the purpuras are bleeding into the skin and bleeding from the mucous membranes.

TABLE 3

A simplified 'bird's-eye view' of the pathogenesis of some common and commonly talked about haemorrhagic diseases. The platelet defects indicated are quantitative (thrombocytopenia) except in Glanzmann's and Von Willebrand's disease where they are qualitative. There may be a qualitative platelet defect in scurvy also.

The haemorrhagic diseases	Clotting defect	Platelet defect	Vessel defect
Haemophilia	yes	—	—
Christmas disease	yes	—	—
PTA deficiency	yes	—	—
Prothrombin deficiency	yes	—	—
Fibrinogen deficiency	yes	—	—
Factor V deficiency	yes	—	—
Factor VII deficiency	yes	—	—
Werlhof's disease	—	yes	—
Acute leukaemia	—	yes	—
Aplastic anaemia	—	yes	—
Megaloblastic anaemia	—	yes	—
Lupus erythematosis	—	yes	—
Glanzmann's disease	—	yes	—
Henoch–Schönlein disease	—	—	yes
Senile purpura	—	—	yes
Scurvy	—	—	yes
Hereditary telangiectasia	—	—	yes
Ehlers–Danlos syndrome	—	—	yes
Moschcowitz's syndrome	—	yes	yes
Von Willebrand's disease	yes	yes	yes

Notwithstanding the clinical usefulness of this classification, the student is warned that he will not infrequently find it defective. Sometimes, for example, a haemorrhagic disease will be seen which will fit into both categories and, indeed, sometimes one which will fit into neither. Such is the way with most classifications in medicine. The clinician's first job is done when he recognizes the haemorrhagic nature of the disease. This he does by the criteria laid down on page 73. It is for the laboratory then to take the matter further. In the light of the laboratory reports the case is reviewed.

THE CLOTTING DISEASES

The following are the more important clotting diseases.

Haemophilia

Haemophilia is due to a deficiency of antihaemophilic factor, a deficiency which is genetically determined. For practical purposes it may be said that it occurs only in males; this shows that the gene is sex-linked. The outstanding clinical feature is haemarthrosis which is often crippling in its effect, but repeated haemorrhage, following mild or even unnoticed trauma, from practically any site is common. Prolonged bleeding after circumcision, tonsillectomy, or tooth extraction often brings the case to light in the first place. Should bleeding or oozing of blood persist for 24 hours after any of these operations, mild suspicion is aroused; should it continue for 48 hours, grave suspicion is aroused. Haematomas, often painful and sometimes dangerous because of their position, are not uncommon and sometimes haematuria with renal colic is the most prominent feature.

The blood findings are interesting because they show so few pathological changes. The whole blood clotting time is typically increased, as would be expected, yet almost 50 per cent of cases have a normal whole blood clotting time. A far more sensitive test is the partial thromboplastin time (PTT), which is therefore the test of choice in preliminary investigations. The prothrombin time is normal. This combination of a prolonged PTT and a normal prothrombin index (PI) places the defect in the first phase of the clotting mechanism and in more than 90 per cent of cases it will prove to be haemophilia. The differential PTT will distinguish the defects of the first phase.

The blood film is essentially normal (unless there has been significant haemorrhage). The bleeding time is normal as there is no deficiency of platelets or vascular contraction, and the capillary fragility test is normal (*see* Clinical protocol 21).

Christmas disease

Christmas disease is due to a deficiency of Christmas factor. Clinically and genetically it is indistinguishable from haemophilia; it is, however, usually a more mild condition. The distinction between the two can be made in the laboratory by means of the differential PTT.

Plasma thromboplastin antecedent deficiency

Plasma thromboplastin antecedent (PTA) deficiency is also known as Rosenthal's disease. It is similar to both haemophilia and Christmas disease but is determined by a non-sex-linked gene. It is usually brought to light following tooth extraction or tonsillectomy and is distinguished from haemophilia and Christmas disease by the differential PTT.

Factor V deficiency

Factor V deficiency is also known as parahaemophilia or Owren's disease. It occurs in a congenital and an acquired form. The acquired form is associated with a number of conditions, notably liver disease. In these cases, other clotting factors are often deficient as well.

Factor VII deficiency

Factor VII deficiency also occurs in a congenital and acquired form. The acquired defect is often associated with liver disease, but the most common cause of factor VII deficiency is the administration of coumarin drugs, especially ethyl biscoumacetate (Tromexan). These cases sometimes occur as emergencies. The best treatment is a blood (preferably fresh blood) transfusion.

Prothrombin deficiency

Prothrombin deficiency occurs in haemorrhagic disease of the newborn when it is usually associated with deficiencies of factors VII and X. The haemorrhage, which may be from the umbilicus, the nose, the stomach or the vagina, usually starts in the first few days of life. Treatment is by transfusion of fresh blood. Vitamin K may be helpful in some cases.

Fibrinogen deficiency

Fibrinogen deficiency may occur in a congenital or acquired form. The acquired form, which is by far the more common, is associated with a number of conditions, notably obstetrical disorders and liver disease. Treatment is by plasma or blood transfusion. Concentrates are available as well.

Circulating anticoagulants

Rarely, substances appear in the blood which inhibit the action of certain clotting factors. Though they are all rare, the most common is one which inhibits antihaemophilic factor. Their presence should be suspected when a patient with a known clotting factor deficiency does not respond favourably when the appropriate factor is administered in blood, plasma or serum.

The laboratory investigation of a clotting disease

Because of the great number of tests which have been recommended from time to time, the student is likely to be confused when faced with the investigation of a clotting defect. The situation is worsened because some of these tests are crude (for example, the whole blood clotting time) and therefore positively misleading. The following is offered as a highly simplified approach to the problem. Though simple, it will nevertheless cater for the vast majority of cases.

A haemorrhagic disease having been recognized at the bedside (by the criteria given on page 73), and a clotting defect being suspected, a specimen of blood is sent to the laboratory for the following tests.

(1) Partial thromboplastin time (PTT).
(2) Prothrombin time.
(3) Differential partial thromboplastin time.

Interpretation of the results

(1) A prolonged PTT, in association with a normal prothrombin time, indicates a defect in the first phase of the clotting mechanism. In more than 90 per cent of cases the defect will turn out to be either haemophilia or Christmas disease.
(2) The differential partial thromboplastin test will distinguish between the defects of the first phase.
(3) A prolonged PTT, in association with a prolonged prothrombin time, will indicate a defect in the second or third phase of the clotting mechanism. In the majority of cases, it will be due to overdosage with coumarin drugs, but it may be due to haemorrhagic disease of the newborn or fibrinogen deficiency. The clinical history of the case will go far in resolving the problem, but it may be necessary to employ more specific tests.
(4) A normal PTT in association with a normal prothrombin time excludes any significant defect in the clotting mechanism.

Clinical protocol 21.   Haemophilia

A man aged 18 years was admitted to hospital because of a painful swollen right knee joint. On examination it had the appearance of a haemarthrosis; furthermore, there was strong evidence of a previous haemarthrosis in the left knee joint.

Haemogram

Haemoglobin	7·9 g%	White cell count	7,000/mm³
		Neutrophils	70%
PCV	27%	Monocytes	4%
		Lymphocytes	23%
MCHC	29%	Eosinophils	3%
		Basophils	0%

The red cells are hypochromic and microcytic; they show anisocytosis and occasional polychromatic forms. The white cells are normal. The platelets are normal in number and appearance.

Comment

The clinical picture is suggestive of a clotting defect of which the commonest is haemophilia. The blood picture suggests iron deficiency anaemia due to chronic haemorrhage, dietary deficiency, or a combination of both.

Preliminary coagulation studies revealed a prolonged PTT. This confirmed the presence of a clotting defect. The prothrombin time was normal, hence the defect was placed in the first phase of the clotting mechanism. The differential partial thromboplastin test pin-pointed the condition as haemophilia.

This patient is therefore lacking in three blood factors: iron, red cells and antihaemophilic factor. The best way of supplying all three is by a transfusion of fresh blood. Had the patient not been anaemic, then fresh or freshly frozen plasma or cryoprecipitate would have been a better treatment. In some centres, treatment is controlled by assays of the serum antihaemophilic factor, but where this facility is not available one must depend on clinical observations and ordinary coagulation tests after giving a reasonable dose of the blood product. Finding and keeping suitable employment is the greatest problem facing this patient, and in this matter he should be helped as much as possible. Should further joint haemorrhage occur, he must be treated immediately with AHF in some form or another.

THE PURPURAS

Purpura is such an important sign in clinical medicine that it deserves a special section, which it is now about to receive. Purpura results from haemorrhage into the skin. It varies in appearance from tiny petechial haemorrhages at the one extreme, to large patches of ecchymosis at the other. It varies in significance from the most trivial diseases (purpura simplex) to the most serious (meningococcal septicaemia, haemorrhagic smallpox, typhus fever and others). Because of this, it is a sign which must never be regarded lightly. Here we shall consider only those non-urgent cases in which purpura is among the main clinical presentations and which presents a problem in diagnosis.

By tradition, purpura is subdivided into two groups: thrombocytopenic purpura and non-thrombocytopenic purpura. This division is the first and most logical step in reaching the ultimate diagnosis in problem cases (*see* Table 4).

The diagnosis of thrombocytopenic purpura

Few doctors, even the most experienced, approach this problem without a certain trepidation; such is the extent of the difficulties. The following simplified approach, though not comprehensive, is offered in the hope that it will help and encourage the younger man.

Consider Table 4. Numbers 1, 2, 3, 4 and 5 have a characteristic blood picture, therefore a blood count should be done in all cases. It is important to remember that the blood picture in Werlhof's disease is, apart from the thrombocytopenia, essentially normal. That is what is characteristic about it. Hence, if any other abnormality is found, except such anaemia as might be accounted for by the haemorrhage,

TABLE 4
Thrombocytopenic Purpura

---

(1) Primary thrombocytopenic purpura or Werlhof's disease
(2) Acute leukaemia
(3) Chronic leukaemia
(4) Aplastic anaemia
(5) Megaloblastic anaemia
(6) Lupus erythematosus
(7) Myelofibrosis
(8) Thrombotic thrombocytopenic purpura or Moschcowitz's disease
(9) Drugs
(10) Rarely Felty's syndrome, Gaucher's disease, sarcoidosis and so on.

---

then a cause other than Werlhof's disease must be sought. Numbers 6, 7 and 8 may have a suggestive blood picture. Lupus erythematosus (LE) may easily be confused with Werlhof's disease, but the test for LE cells will often expose it. Myelofibrosis will require a bone marrow examination for diagnosis. Thrombotic thrombocytopenic purpura is usually associated with a haemolytic anaemia of the micro-angiopathic type and a bizarre clinical picture which includes many neurological, and seemingly mental symptoms. The diagnosis of thrombocytopenia due to drugs depends primarily on a history of drug-taking.

Clinical protocols illustrating acute leukaemia, chronic lymphatic leukaemia, aplastic anaemia and myelofibrosis have been given on pages 66, 69, 48 and 57 respectively. Although the cases presented did not in fact have purpura, they did have thrombocytopenia and might well have had purpura. They may therefore be reviewed at this point.

Now follow Clinical protocols 22, 23 and 24. These illustrate Werlhof's disease, the purpura of megaloblastic anaemia and thrombotic thrombocytopenic purpura.

Clinical protocol 22.   Werlhof's disease

A girl aged 15 years was admitted to hospital because of purpura on the arms and legs. A few days previously she had what seemed to be a severe cold, but now, apart from the rash, she appeared to be quite healthy. In particular, there was no enlargement of the spleen. Examination of the stools and urine showed the presence of blood in each.

Haemogram

Haemoglobin	12·3 g%	White cell count	11,000/mm³
		Neutrophils	44%
PCV	36%	Monocytes	7%
		Lymphocytes	49%
MCHC	34%	Eosinophils	0%
		Basophils	0%

The red cells are normochromic and normocytic, and they are otherwise normal in appearance. There is a slight lymphocytosis. The platelets are greatly reduced in number.

Comment

This case illustrates Werlhof's disease, otherwise known as primary thrombocytopenic purpura, and it is probably as 'typical' as one is likely to encounter. On clinical examination it might have passed for purpura simplex, but the reduction of platelet numbers immediately places the condition in the thrombocytopenic group. Furthermore, bleeding into the bowel and urine is not expected in purpura simplex.

In its clinical and haematological aspects, Werlhof's disease may be regarded as a disease of 'negative' features. Clinically, apart from the purpura (and perhaps other haemorrhagic features), there is little to be found. Although the spleen may be slightly enlarged, any moderate or marked enlargement must suggest an alternative condition. Haematologically, apart from the thrombocytopenia (and such changes as might result from the usually trivial haemorrhage), there is little of note. Should other pathological changes be found, an alternative condition is once again suggested. (The lymphocytosis in this case may have been due to the cold). It is this strange 'negative' character of the disease which sets it apart and at the same time makes it a completely unsatisfactory clinical concept. This state of affairs will continue until we know more of its aetiology.

Clinical protocol 23.   Megaloblastic anaemia

An infant aged 11 months was brought to hospital because of pallor and purpura. The purpuric rash was distributed all over the body. There was no sternal tenderness, no enlargement of the spleen and no history of drug-taking.

Haemogram

Haemoglobin	4·2 g%	White cell count	10,000/mm³
		Neutrophils	39%
PCV	12%	Monocytes	7%
		Lymphocytes	54%
MCHC	35%	Eosinophils	0%
		Basophils	0%

The red cells are normochromic and macrocytic; they show marked anisocytosis, marked poikilocytosis, increased diffuse polychromasia, punctate basophilia and occasional nucleated forms. Among the white cells, occasional giant myeloid forms were seen. The platelets are markedly reduced in number.

Comment

Occasionally purpura is among the more prominent features in patients with megaloblastic anaemia. Although megaloblasts were not demonstrated in the peripheral blood in this case, the haemogram is so highly suggestive that most doctors would probably be prepared to accept this as a case of megaloblastic anaemia of infancy. If absolute proof were necessary, one could resort to bone marrow examination, but such a procedure seemed unnecessary in this patient. Having accepted the case as megaloblastic anaemia, we may also reasonably presume that it is due to folic acid deficiency. Here again, should absolute proof be required, one would estimate the folic acid content of the patient's serum. A final reasonable assumption is that the folic acid deficiency is a manifestation of malnutrition.

As malnutrition is seldom specific, the treatment of the patient consists in correcting the diet and supplementing it with folic acid. It would be wise also to add the other vitamins, especially vitamin B_{12} and vitamin C.

As three assumptions were made, it is necessary to follow the effects of the treatment. The baby's weight and haemoglobin concentration should be checked at weekly intervals. If the expected response is not obtained, then the aetiology of the condition should be reviewed.

Clinical protocol 24.   Thrombotic thrombocytopenic purpura

A man aged 30 years was admitted to hospital in a state of mental confusion. Sometimes he was drowsy, and at other times he was exceedingly restless. He was unable to speak, yet at times he seemed to be able to understand the spoken word. On examination, generalized purpura was discovered. There was no enlargement of the lymphatic glands or spleen and there was no sternal tenderness.

Haemogram

Haemoglobin	6·3 g%	White cell count	9,000/mm³
		Neutrophils	80%
PCV	18%	Monocytes	4%
		Lymphocytes	15%
MCHC	35%	Eosinophils	1%
		Basophils	0%

The red cells are normochromic and normocytic; they show marked anisocytosis and extreme poikilocytosis. Among the poikilocytes are burr cells, helmet cells, triangular cells and cells the shape of which is beyond description. In addition, there are spherocytes and polychromatic cells. There is a slight lymphopenia. The platelets are markedly reduced in number (13,000/mm³.

Comment

Had it not been for the discovery of the purpura in this case, the patient might well have been referred to a psychiatrist. But the purpura demanded a blood count and this immediately put an entirely different complexion on the case. The haemogram reveals the typical picture of micro-angiopathic haemolytic anaemia, and at once the bizarre clinical picture is exposed as thrombotic thrombocytopenic purpura, otherwise known as Moschcowitz's disease. Our knowledge of the pathogenesis of the condition is scanty. The essential pathological change is the occurrence of occluding lesions in arterioles and capillaries throughout the body, especially in the heart and brain. Of the origin and nature of these lesions we know practically nothing, but they seemingly lead to the most *outré* effects which constitute the clinical and haematological manifestations of this strange and fatal disease.

There is no satisfactory treatment. Steroid hormones may be tried and blood transfusions may be given if required. The prognosis is hopeless; death may be expected within a few weeks.

Non-thrombocytopenic purpura

However difficult the diagnosis of thrombocytopenic purpura, the non-thrombocytopenic group presents an even greater problem. In this group, the clinician must depend more on his own resources as little help is forthcoming from the laboratory (*see* Table 5).

TABLE 5
Non-thrombocytopenic Purpura

Purpura simplex
Senile purpura
Hereditary haemorrhagic telangiectasia
Von Willebrand's disease
Henoch–Schönlein's purpura
Ehlers–Danlos syndrome
Scurvy
Polycythaemia vera
Myelomatosis
Glanzmann's disease
Haemorrhagic thrombocythaemia
Drugs
A variety of acute infections
Chronic renal, liver and heart diseases

Purpura simplex

The patient is usually a woman of childbearing age who complains of easy bruising. The patient feels perfectly well but sometimes complains of menorrhagia. This condition, although disfiguring, is harmless.

Senile purpura

Senile purpura is a common condition in persons over 60 years of age. The purpuric patches appear characteristically on the dorsum of the hands and the extensor surfaces of the forearms. Like purpura simplex, the condition is disfiguring but harmless.

Hereditary haemorrhagic telangiectasia

Bleeding from the mucous membranes, rather than purpura, is more characteristic of this condition. Usually the telangiectases are visible on the lips, the roof of the mouth, the nasal cavity, or the face. But they may be present in areas where they cannot be seen. The disease is inherited by a simple dominant gene.

Von Willebrand's disease

Von Willebrand's disease has a strong claim to be included among the clotting defects rather than among the purpuras. Patients usually present with a complaint of prolonged bleeding after minor trauma. Epistaxis is common. One of my patients bled for days after an intramuscular injection.

Henoch–Schönlein's disease

Henoch–Schönlein's disease is seen mainly in children. The distribution of the rash is symmetrical and it is located mainly on the limbs and buttocks. The rash is often preceded by an upper respiratory infection which occurs 1–3 weeks previously, and it is often accompanied by painful swellings of the joints and abdominal colic.

The Ehlers–Danlos syndrome

The Ehlers–Danlos syndrome is distinguished by a remarkable hyperextensibility of joints. There is also a tendency for scar tissue to stretch and for pouches of skin to form about the knee and elbow joints. It is inherited by a simple dominant gene.

Scurvy

The purpuric rash of scurvy occurs typically on the legs. In addition there may be bleeding from the mucous membranes, painful haematomas and other signs, not only of vitamin C deficiency but of malnutrition in general.

Polycythaemia vera

Purpura occurs in some cases of polycythaemia vera but it is seldom a prominent complaint. The blood count will solve the problem in these cases.

Myelomatosis

Haemorrhagic manifestations including purpura are not uncommon in patients with myelomatosis. The diagnosis of this condition is discussed on page 72.

Glanzmann's disease

This is a rare condition which is due to a functional defect of the platelets. The platelets are normal in number, but abnormal in appearance. Giant platelets are commonly seen.

Hereditary thrombocythaemia

In this rare condition there is an excessive number of platelets, but the platelets are often abnormal in function and appearance. Many patients with this condition have an atrophy or an absence of the spleen.

Drugs

The drugs which are associated with non-thrombocytopenia are listed in Table 10, page 91.

Clinical protocol 25.   Henoch–Schönlein's purpura

A boy aged 7 years was admitted to hospital because of abdominal pain and vomiting. On examination he was found to have a purpuric rash on the limbs, soles of the feet and buttocks. There was no history of infection, drug-taking or abnormal mental conduct; there was no sternal tenderness or enlargement of the spleen.

Haemogram

Haemoglobin	13·8 g%	White cell count	11,000/mm³
		Neutrophils	55%
PCV	40%	Monocytes	7%
		Lymphocytes	37%
MCHC	34%	Eosinophils	1%
		Basophils	0%

The red cells are normochromic and normocytic. There is a slight lymphocytosis. The platelets are normal in number and appearance.

Comment

This, if ever there was one, is a classical example of Henoch–Schönlein's purpura. The haemogram immediately excludes Werlhof's disease and all the other forms of thrombocytopenic purpura, while the clinical history, in the light of the haemogram, can hardly be explained by anything other than Henoch–Schönlein's purpura.

The condition is due to capillary damage, which itself is probably due to an allergic reaction. Like rheumatic fever and acute nephritis, it often follows an upper respiratory infection. Such a history, however, was not obtained in this case.

The abdominal pain and vomiting suggest an acute abdominal emergency but the skin rash, which is always present, and the joint pain, which is often present, make a fairly easily recognizable clinical picture.

The treatment consists essentially in bed rest; many patients require nothing more. Steroid hormones were given to this patient who recovered in about 1 week. One wonders how long it would have taken had he not received the hormones.

A slight lymphocytosis is noted in the haemogram. The absolute lymphocyte count is just over 4,000, while the upper limit of normality is 3,500. This is insignificant.

Clinical protocol 26. Hereditary haemorrhagic telangiectasia

A man aged 40 years was admitted to hospital because of spontaneous bleeding from the nose and mouth. Similar attacks occurred intermittently over a period of some 10 years or more. Recently the attacks had become more severe. On questioning, the patient also admitted to loss of energy and excessive tiredness.

Haemogram

Haemoglobin	10·6 g%	White cell count	7,000/mm³
		Neutrophils	59%
PCV	35%	Monocytes	8%
		Lymphocytes	33%
MCHC	30%	Eosinophils	0%
		Basophils	0%

The red cells are normocytic and slightly hypochromic; they show anisocytosis and cigar-shaped poikilocytes. In addition, there is increased diffuse polychromasia. The white cells are normal in appearance. The platelets are normal in number and appearance.

Comment

Hereditary haemorrhagic telangiectasia is determined by a simple Mendelian dominant gene. It therefore attacks both sexes equally. Though an inherited condition, it often does not become manifest until puberty or even adulthood; furthermore, as it seems to skip generations from time to time, a clear history of its inheritance is not always forthcoming.

The most common clinical feature of the disease is bleeding from the nose, but there may be bleeding from the mouth, the respiratory, the gastro-intestinal or the genito-urinary systems. The bleeding eventually leads to the anaemia of chronic haemorrhage.

The diagnosis of the condition depends on finding the typical telangiectases. When these are on the skin or the lips they are immediately apparent; more often they are in the nasal cavity or the roof of the mouth where they are still easily seen. If they are elsewhere they may not be demonstrable.

Treatment is directed towards the control of the bleeding and the replacement of the lost iron. Electrocauterization of the nasal septum and the turbinates is often resorted to. Blood transfusion may be required for the anaemia. Although included here, there is no clotting defect and no defect in the platelets.

9—Drug-induced Disorders of the Blood

The number of different disorders of the blood that can be caused by drugs and the number of different drugs that can cause disorders of the blood are quite frightening. Furthermore, the latter is growing. Drugs may cause anaemia of various kinds (aplastic, haemolytic and megaloblastic), purpura (both thrombocytopenic and non-thrombocytopenic), agranulocytosis and methaemoglobinaemia. This is why it is so important, in the course of taking the clinical history, to question the patient specifically on any medicines which he may have been taking. In this connection it is better to use the word 'medicine' rather than 'drug' as the latter carries an unsavoury, if not a criminal, connotation these days.

WARNING SIGNS AND EMERGENCY TREATMENT

There are a few warning signs of drug toxicity with which the doctor should be familiar. If, in the course of treatment, self-administered or administered by the doctor himself, a patient develops any of the following signs, then the presence of haematological poisoning must be suspected and the treatment revised with this in mind. The signs are: (1) anaemia, (2) sore throat with fever (agranulocytosis), and (3) purpura.

Every drug the patient has been taking must be checked for its toxic potentialities. The manufacturer's enclosure is often helpful in this matter but, in addition, tables of the more important and commonly used drugs, together with the diseases they cause, are given in this chapter. Should suspicion fall on a particular drug it must be discontinued immediately. In most cases a satisfactory substitute can be found.

THE DRUGS AND THE DISEASES

The following tables are not intended to be exhaustive. The drugs mentioned have been selected not only because of their toxic potentialities but also because of their popularity. For the sake of brevity, those drugs with toxic effects which are in fact the desired therapeutic effect have been omitted.

TABLE 6

Drugs which cause anaemia (aplastic), neutropenia and thrombocytopenia

Drug	Anaemia	Neutropenia	Thrombocytopenia
Choramphenicol	yes	yes	yes
Streptomycin	yes	yes	yes
Sulphonamides	yes	yes	yes
Tolbutamide	yes	yes	yes
Methoin (Mesantoin)	yes	yes	yes
Paramethadione	yes	yes	yes
Troxidone	yes	yes	yes
Phenylbutazone	yes	yes	yes
Isoniazid	yes	yes	yes
Chlorpromazine	yes	yes	yes
Gold	yes	yes	yes
Amidopyrine	—	yes	—
Thiouracil	—	yes	—
Dicoumarol	—	yes	—
PAS	—	yes	—
Quinine	—	—	yes
Quinidine	—	—	yes
Sedormid	—	—	yes
Acetazolamide	—	—	yes
Chlorpropamide	—	—	yes

TABLE 7

Drugs which cause haemolytic anaemia in G-6-PD deficiency and those which cause it by means of an immune mechanism

Drug	G-6-PD deficiency	Immune mechanism
Chloroquin	yes	—
Primaquine	yes	—
Pentaquin	yes	—
Quinacrine	yes	—
Acetylsalicylic acid	yes	—
Chloramphenicol	yes	—
Sulphoxone	yes	—
Quinine	yes	yes
Quinidine	yes	yes
Phenacetin	yes	yes
Sulphonamides	yes	yes
PAS	yes	yes
Penicillin	—	yes
Stibophen	—	yes
Methyldopa	—	yes

TABLE 8
Drugs known to cause megaloblastic anaemia

Phenytoin	(anticonvulsant)
Primidone	(anticonvulsant)
Methotrexate	(cancer chemotherapy)
Cytosine arabinoside	(cancer chemotherapy)

Should megaloblastic anaemia occur in the course of treating epilepsy, folic acid should be given.

TABLE 9
Drugs which cause methaemoglobinaemia

Nitrites
Nitrates
Sulphonamides
Phenacetin
Acetanilide

Methaemoglobin is constantly being formed in normal circumstances but it is rapidly reduced to haemoglobin. It is believed that these drugs overwhelm the reducing mechanism with the result that methaemoglobinaemia, which leads to cyanosis, occurs. Young infants are particularly susceptible.

TABLE 10
Drugs sometimes associated with non-thrombocytopenic purpura

Iodides
Atropine
Quinine
Phenacetin
Salicylic acid
Chloral hydrate

10—Blood Groups and Transfusion

With the establishment of blood banks in all the large centres and indeed in many primitive areas, the importance of a knowledge of blood groups to the clinician is diminishing. Nevertheless, as he is ultimately responsible for the welfare of the patient, the basic principles, at least should be known. These will be discussed here. Further details of the serology of blood groups will be found in *A Primer of Immunology* (Ward, 1970).

Before the blood of one person may be transfused into another it must be compatible. What is meant by 'compatible'? Compatible, as used here, has two distinct meanings or implications, as follows.

(1) The donor red cells must not react with antibody already present in the recipient's plasma.

(2) The donor cells must not stimulate the production of antibodies in the recipient's plasma.

The first requirement

The first and most important of these requirements is satisfied by doing a pre-transfusion cross-matching test, wherein the red cells of the proposed donor are mixed under suitable conditions with the serum of the recipient. After a period of incubation, the mixture is examined for agglutination, haemolysis and sensitization. If it is done properly, this test requires about an hour to complete. If short cuts are taken, risks are introduced, but on occasions these risks are justified.

The second requirement

This requirement is the most difficult to understand. We can say at once that it is never completely satisfied, but it is sufficiently satisfied for practical purposes by grouping the recipient and the donor in regard to ABO and Rh_0 and selecting the appropriate group for the cross-matching test.

The risk

From what has been said about the second requirement, it will be apparent that, even if there is no technical or clerical error, there will, nevertheless, be a risk. It is perhaps an impertinence to lay down what risks other people should take, so I shall illustrate the point by speaking for myself and taking my own blood group as an example.

I am group A, Rh positive. Should I need a transfusion I would be perfectly happy to receive donor blood which was group A, Rh positive, provided a cross-matching test was done; this is probably exactly what I would get. Now consider the risk I would be taking. I said I was group A, Rh positive; that is correct, but more precisely I am group A_2, Rh_1 Rh_1. The donor blood, on the other hand, would probably be group A_1, Rh rh. In other words, I would be receiving at least two foreign blood factors, A_1, and hr^1 in the ABO and Rh systems alone. This says nothing of the MN, Kell, Duffy, Kidd and so on, factors which I would be receiving and which might be foreign to me. Clearly I would be better off with group O, rh blood*, but I would gladly accept the other because the chances of my suffering from it are probably far less than the chance of my being killed while driving to work. That is a chance I accept every morning with hardly a thought. But were I a woman with ambitions of raising a family I might not be so agreeable, especially if the transfusion was not really necessary.

Other sources of danger

Far more important than the above is the risk of giving the wrong blood to a patient. This may arise for a number of reasons, the most common of which are not technical but clerical.

(1) Blood for compatibility testing may be collected from patient Smith but inadvertently labelled with the name of patient Jones. When the donor blood arrives from the blood bank it will be marked as suitable for patient Jones for whom it may in fact prove fatal. Great care must therefore be taken in both collecting and labelling.

(2) Donor blood intended for Mr. A. Smith may, especially if there is an element of urgency, be given to Mr. B. Smith. It is therefore not sufficient to label the specimen with the patient's name; the patient's hospital number should be included. This will subsequently appear on the container of donor blood and should be checked before giving the transfusion. Checking numbers, especially long numbers, is a tedious business when a transfusion is required; but it never seems so tedious in the chilly atmosphere of the inquest room.

* O, rh is the so-called Universal doner blood.

The use of the appropriate product

It is good practice as well as good economy to use the appropriate product, whole blood or packed red cells, whenever a transfusion is required. Experience alone will tell which ought to be administered to a given patient, but broadly speaking packed cells are not used as often as they ought to be. Most 'medical' anaemias, for example, require only packed cells if a transfusion is required at all. To give whole blood, which contains about 60 per cent plasma, is not only redundant, it limits the volume which may be given at a time.

The ordering of blood

As a rough guide it may be said that a half litre of blood, or the packed cells obtained from a half litre of blood, will raise the haemoglobin level of the average adult (weight 70 kilos) by about 1 g per cent. From this, the amount of blood required can be calculated and thus the order is sent to the blood bank. However, the volume of blood administered to the patient must be decided, not by a mathematical calculation but by clinical observation of the patient.

The issuing of blood by the blood bank

As a general rule blood banks provide a service the safety of which is adjusted to meet the urgency of the case. These degrees of safety may be considered under three headings.

(1) If the case is a desperate emergency the blood may be issued without any pre-transfusion testing. As the blood in these circumstances will be of the rather rare group O, Rh-negative type, this facility should not be requested unless the case really is a desperate emergency. If an incompatibility results, which it may, the onus will be on the person who ordered the blood to justify his request.

(2) Blood may be issued on 'emergency compatibility testing'. In this routine, certain short cuts are taken in the blood bank and the blood can be made available in about 20 minutes. As stated before, this decrease in time involves an increase in risk, and should an untoward reaction occur the clinician may have to justify his request before a magistrate.

(3) Blood may be, and usually is, issued on a 'standard' compatibility procedure. This is the safest way of issuing blood but involves a Coombs test which itself requires about 1 hour to do. If a reaction occurs following this procedure, it is unlikely that a magistrate will find anyone negligent.

UNTOWARD REACTIONS FOLLOWING TRANSFUSION

A number of untoward reactions may follow blood transfusion. They include haemolytic reactions, allergic reactions, heart failure with pulmonary oedema, febrile reactions, infection, clotting defects, haemosiderosis and thrombophlebitis. Only the more important of these, either because of their frequency or special danger, will be considered here.

Haemolytic transfusion reactions

Haemolytic tranfusion reactions follow the use of the wrong blood, the use of time-expired blood, or the use of accidentally over-heated or frozen blood. The circumstances in which these occur automatically suggest the means of preventing them.

The clinical manifestations of a haemolytic reaction vary greatly. They may be hardly perceptible, there may be pyrexia, rigors, pains in the back and limbs and oliguria progressing to anuria, or there may be sudden collapse and death. As soon as it is suspected that a haemolytic reaction is taking place, the transfusion should be discontinued and the patient should be placed on an intake–output chart. A specimen of the patient's blood and the remains of the donor blood should be returned to the blood bank for checking. If a gross incompatibility is discovered the treatment of the patient will probably be that of acute renal shut-down.

Allergic reactions

Allergic reactions are due to an antigen in the donor blood to which the patient is hypersensitive. They therefore cannot be detected by the blood bank beforehand. They usually take the form of urticaria, swellings of the face, erythematous rashes and sometimes bronchial asthma. In the majority of cases the attack is trivial but sometimes it is quite severe. Because of their frequency, some practitioners administer antihistamine to all patients before transfusion, others administer it only to those who have a history of allergy. If given at all, it should be given to the patient and not injected into the container of donor blood. The attack can usually be controlled with adrenaline.

Heart failure with pulmonary oedema

Heart failure with pulmonary oedema is due to overloading of the circulation and is probably the greatest single danger of blood transfusion today. It therefore behoves the practitioner to be aware of the early signs so that treatment can be started immediately. When these signs are detected, the first thing to do is to stop the transfusion and prop the patient up in bed. If there is no improvement after 5 or 10 minutes then a half litre of blood should be withdrawn; this may be repeated if necessary. Finally, the standard treatment for acute heart failure may be required.

The incidence of this complication can be reduced by giving smaller volume and giving it at a slower rate. In 'medical' cases, it is broadly true to say that the more severe the anaemia, the less blood should be given and the slower it should be given. The use of packed cells, rather than whole blood, will also reduce the over-all frequency of the condition.

Virus hepatitis

Although a few different kinds of infections may result from blood transfusion,* the most important by far is virus hepatitis. It is important, not only because it is such a severe disease, but also because of its high frequency. It is said to follow about 1 per cent of whole blood transfusions and up to 20 per cent of pooled serum transfusions.† In addition, it may result from the administration of such blood products as albumen, fibrinogen, cryoprecipitate and others.

Recently it has been suggested that the Australian antigen may prove of value in screening blood donors with a view to excluding carriers of the virus of hepatitis. At the present time there is no satisfactory way of doing so, nor is there any way of sterilizing blood or blood products in regard to this virus.

There is, however, a possibility that the disease may be prevented by the use of human gamma-globulin as a passive immunizing agent. This, of course, carries the risk of transmitting the very disease which it is given to prevent. There is no doubt that the incidence of virus hepatitis would be reduced if the use of pooled serum were abandoned.

Citrate intoxication

As citrate is the anticoagulant used as a routine by blood banks, the question of citrate intoxication arises. The danger, in fact, is very small and is seen almost exclusively in only two circumstances: during exchange transfusion in infants and when massive transfusions of blood are given. In infants, muscle tremors and prolongation of the ST segment in the electrocardiogram have been noted and are attributed to the citrate. For this reason many practitioners give a prophylactic dose of 10 per cent calcium gluconate in the course of the transfusion.

* Malaria, syphilis, brucellosis.
† 20 per cent is 1 in 5, so you have a better chance in Russian roulette.

When massive transfusions are anticipated, for example, in open heart operations, the donor blood should be collected in heparin rather than in citrate; thus the complication is avoided. It might reasonably be asked why donor blood is not collected in heparin as a routine. The reason is because blood collected in heparin cannot be stored for more than 24 hours, hence if blood for all transfusions were collected in this way there would inevitably be a great wastage.

Transfusion siderosis

We have already seen how difficult it is to absorb iron; it is far more difficult to excrete it. Hence, any iron administered parenterally (a half litre of blood contains 250 mg of iron) is retained by the body and, for all practical purposes, can only be removed by bleeding. In patients who require repeated transfusions and who are not bleeding (for example, patients with aplastic anaemia), excessive deposits of iron may occur in the liver and this might lead to fibrosis. The danger, however, does not arise until a great many transfusions (possibly 50 litres of blood) are given.

Test Questions

CHAPTER 1

1. How do you define 'anaemia'?
2. Discuss the importance of individual normality in regard to haemoglobin concentration.
3. Discuss the importance of fluid balance in regard to haemoglobin concentration.
4. How is anaemia recognized in the laboratory?
5. Give the morphological classification of anaemia.
6. Name the findings on the blood film which are of importance in diagnosis.
7. Name the three pathogenetic mechanisms of anaemia. Discuss briefly the importance of each.
8. Discuss the multifactorial origin of anaemia.
9. Discuss erythropoiesis in anaemia.
10. How is megaloblastic erythropoiesis suspected, strongly suspected and definitely recognized from an examination of the blood film?

CHAPTER 2

1. What are the three points about acute haemorrhage which are often overlooked?
2. Describe the blood picture in acute haemorrhage.
3. Describe the blood picture in chronic haemorrhage.
4. With which conditions may the blood picture in chronic haemorrhage be confused?
5. Outline the treatment of chronic haemorrhage.

CHAPTER 3

1. What is the essence of haemolytic anaemia?
2. Discuss the catabolism of haemoglobin.
3. Discuss the fate of free haemoglobin in the plasma.
4. What compensatory phenomena occur in haemolytic anaemia?
5. Discuss the clinical diagnosis of haemolytic anaemia.
6. Describe the blood picture in haemolytic anaemia.
7. Discuss the importance of the family history in patients with haemolytic anaemia.

8. Describe the inheritance of hereditary spherocytosis.
9. Describe the inheritance of sickle cell anaemia.
10. Name the causes of haemolytic anaemia.
11. Which iso-antibodies commonly cause haemolytic anaemia?
12. Write a note on auto-allergic haemolytic anaemia.
13. What is meant by 'micro-angiopathic haemolytic anaemia'? With what conditions is it associated?
14. What is meant by 'myelophthisic anaemia'? What are the causes of myelophthisic anaemia?
15. Describe the blood picture in micro-angiopathic haemolytic anaemia.
16. Describe the clinical and blood pictures in Mediterranean anaemia.
17. Discuss the clinical diagnosis of hereditary spherocytosis.
18. Describe the blood picture in hereditary spherocytosis.
19. Discuss the treatment of hereditary spherocytosis.
20. Discuss the line of thought which leads to the diagnosis of sickle cell anaemia.

CHAPTER 4

1. What are the causes of marrow failure?
2. Discuss the diagnosis of marrow failure.
3. What is meant by 'megaloblastic anaemia'?
4. Describe the blood picture in megaloblastic anaemia.
5. What is meant by 'the anaemia of general malnutrition'?
6. What is the relationship between malnutrition, infection and anaemia?
7. Discuss the aetiology of general malnutrition.
8. Describe the blood pictures which may occur in general malnutrition.
9. What do you understand by 'iron deficiency anaemia'?
10. Discuss the aetiology of nutritional iron deficiency anaemia.
11. Name the important sources of iron in the diet.
12. Describe the clinical features of nutritional iron deficiency anaemia.
13. Discuss the treatment of nutritional iron deficiency anaemia.
14. What are the important sources of folic acid in the diet?
15. Folic acid is heat-labile. What is the practical importance of this fact?
16. In what circumstances in particular is folic acid deficiency likely to occur?
17. Discuss the diagnosis of folic acid deficiency anaemia.
18. Describe the FIGlu excretion test.
19. Write a note on latent folic acid deficiency.
20. What are the important sources of vitamin B_{12} in the diet?
21. Describe the absorption of vitamin B_{12}.
22. In what circumstances is deficiency of vitamin B_{12} likely to occur?
23. What are the clinical effects of vitamin B_{12} deficiency?
24. Discuss the pathogenesis of Addisonian pernicious anaemia.
25. Outline the thought process which leads to the diagnosis of Addisonian pernicious anaemia.
26. What morphological kinds of anaemia occur as a result of infection?

27. How is the hypochromic anaemia of infection distinguished from the hypochromic anaemia of nutritional iron deficiency?
28. Discuss the treatment of the anaemia of infection.
29. Discuss the pathogenesis and aetiology of the anaemia of infection.
30. Discuss the pathogenesis of the anaemia of renal failure.
31. Describe the ways in which drugs may cause anaemia.
32. Describe a typical case of aplastic anaemia. Outline the treatment which might be required.
33. Discuss the morphology, pathogenesis and treatment of the anaemia of hypothyroidism.

CHAPTER 5

1. How would you set about the investigation of a patient with anaemia?
2. What three points in the clinical history must never be forgotten?
3. When requesting a blood count, what information would you supply?
4. If gastro-intestinal haemorrhage is suspected, what further investigations are indicated?
5. Why should the urine be tested in patients with anaemia?
6. Name the anaemias which may have prominent psychological manifestations.

CHAPTER 6

1. Write a note on blood transfusion in the treatment of anaemia.
2. What morphological type of anaemia should be treated with iron?
3. Which kinds of hypochromic anaemia will not respond to iron treatment?
4. What are the indications for folic acid treatment?
5. Why is it important to be reasonably sure of the diagnosis before treating a patient suspected of having pernicious anaemia, with vitamin B_{12}?
6. If a bone marrow examination is to be done, it should be done before vitamin B_{12} or folic acid is administered—why?
7. What is the characteristic feature about the specific treatment of the anaemia of hypothyroidism?
8. What is the indication for the use of pyridoxine?
9. Write a note on splenectomy as a treatment for anaemia.

CHAPTER 7

1. What do you understand by the concept of myeloproliferative disease?
2. Write a note on myelofibrosis.
3. What are the prominent clinical features of chronic myeloid leukaemia?
4. Describe the blood picture in chronic myeloid leukaemia.
5. Discuss the treatment and prognosis of chronic myeloid leukaemia.
6. Discuss the diagnosis of polycythaemia vera.
7. What features in the blood count favour primary rather than secondary polycythaemia?

TEST QUESTIONS

8. What are the main complications of polycythaemia vera?
9. Describe the blood picture in acute leukaemia.
10. What is the most important clinical sign of acute leukaemia?
11. Discuss the treatment and prognosis of acute leukaemia.
12. Describe the blood picture in chronic lymphatic leukaemia.
13. What are the immunological complications of chronic lymphatic leukaemia?
14. Outline the treatment and prognosis in chronic lymphatic leukaemia.
15. What is the commonest clinical feature of myelomatosis?
16. What are the most constant changes in the blood in cases of myelomatosis?
17. How is the diagnosis of myelomatosis usually achieved?
18. Outline the treatment and prognosis of myelomatosis.

CHAPTER 8

1. What are the clinical hall-marks of a haemorrhagic disease?
2. Write a note on the haemostatic mechanism.
3. Write a note on the pathogenesis of the haemorrhagic diseases.
4. Write a note on haemophilia.
5. Outline the initial laboratory investigation of a haemorrhagic disease.
6. Name the common causes of thrombocytopenic purpura.
7. What is the characteristic feature in the blood count in patients with Werlhof's disease?
8. Name the common causes of non-thrombocytopenic purpura.
9. Describe the pathogenesis of hereditary haemorrhagic telangiectasia.
10. How is the diagnosis of hereditary haemorrhagic telangiectasia achieved?

CHAPTER 9

1. Name the kinds of abnormality which may appear in the blood as a result of drug poisoning.
2. What are the warning signs of drug toxicity?
3. What are the toxic effects of chloramphenicol on the blood?
4. What is the pathogenesis of haemolytic anaemia due to drugs?
5. What are the toxic effects of sulphonamides on the blood?
6. What are the toxic effects of streptomycin on the blood?
7. Which drugs may induce megaloblastic anaemia?
8. Which drugs may induce methaemoglobinaemia?

CHAPTER 10

1. What do you understand by 'compatible' blood?
2. What is the purpose of the pre-transfusion cross-matching test?
3. What is the purpose of the pre-transfusion grouping test?
4. What are the common circumstances which result in a patient being transfused with the wrong blood?
5. How do haemolytic transfusion reactions arise?

6. How are haemolytic transfusion reactions recognized?
7. What immediate action should be taken when a haemolytic transfusion reaction is suspected?
8. Describe the clinical features of allergic reactions following blood transfusions.
9. Describe the steps to be taken when circulatory overloading occurs.
10. Discuss the cause and prevention of virus hepatitis following blood transfusion.
11. Write a note on siderosis as a complication of blood transfusion.

Index

Methotrexate in leukaemia, 65
Micro-angiopathy causing haemo-
lytic anaemia, 18, 23
Moschcowitz's disease, 84
Myelofibrosis, 56, 81
Myelomatosis, 69, 86
Myeloproliferative diseases, 55–72

Neutropenia, drug-induced, 90

Owren's disease, 77

Packed cell volume, 2
Parahaemophilia, 77
Partial thromboplastin time, 77, 79
Phosphorus, radioactive, 62
Plasma thromboplastin antecedent
deficiency, 77
Platelet agglutination, 74
Polycythaemia vera, 56, 61, 86
Prednisolone in leukaemia, 65
Pregnancy,
folic acid deficiency in, 37
iron deficiency in, 33, 34
Prostatic carcinoma, 24
Prothrombin deficiency, 78
Pulmonary oedema following blood
transfusion, 95
Purpuras, 80
non-thrombocytopenic, 84, 91
senile, 85
simplex, 85
thrombocytopenic, 80
Pyridoxine in treatment of anaemia,
54

Red cell count, 3
Renal failure, anaemia of, 45
Reticulum cell sarcoma, 18

Rheumatoid arthritis, anaemia of,
45
Rosenthal's disease, 77

Scurvy, 86
Shock in haemorrhage, 6
Siderosis, transfusion, 97
Splenectomy in treatment of anae-
mia, 54
Splenic enlargement,
anaemia, in, 22, 23
hereditary spherocytosis, 25
leukaemia, in, 59, 64, 66, 67, 69
myelofibrosis, in, 57
Sternal tenderness, 65, 66
Stomach, mucosal atrophy, 40

Thrombocytopenia,
drug induced, 90
leukaemia, in, 64, 68
Thrombocytopenic purpura, 80
thrombotic, 83
Thrombocytosis, in acute haemorrhage, 7
Total iron binding capacity, 22, 23,
44
Total iron binding capacity, 22, 34,
44
Tromexan, 78

Venesection, 62
Vincristine, 65
Virus hepatitis, 96
Vitamin B_{12} deficiency, 13, 28, 40,
53
Von Willebrand's disease, 85

Werlhof's disease, 81

Xanthomatosis, 18